Essential Oils And Ancient Medicine

The Beginners Reference Guide for Young, Natural and Healing Living with Aromatherapy

Table of Contents

The following eBook is reproduced below with the goal of providing information that is as accurate and reliable as possible. Regardless, purchasing this eBook can be seen as consent to the fact that both the publisher and the author of this book are in no way experts on the topics discussed within and that any recommendations or suggestions that are made herein are for entertainment purposes only. Professionals should be consulted as needed prior to undertaking any of the action endorsed herein.

This declaration is deemed fair and valid by both the American Bar Association and the Committee of Publishers Association and is legally binding throughout the United States.

Furthermore, the transmission, duplication, or reproduction of any of the following work including specific information will be considered an illegal act irrespective of if it is done electronically or in print. This extends to creating a secondary or tertiary copy of the work or a recorded copy and is only allowed with the express written consent from the Publisher. All additional right reserved.

The information in the following pages is broadly considered a truthful and accurate account of facts and as such, any inattention, use, or misuse of the information in question by the reader will render any resulting actions solely under their purview. There are no scenarios in which the publisher or the original author of this work can be in any fashion deemed liable for any hardship or damages that may befall them after undertaking information described herein.

Additionally, the information in the following pages is intended only for informational purposes and should thus be thought of as universal. As befitting its nature, it is presented without assurance regarding its prolonged validity or interim quality. Trademarks that are mentioned are done without written consent and can in no way be considered an endorsement from the trademark holder.

Introduction

Congratulations on downloading *Essential Oils: Ancient Medicine* and thank you for doing so.

Essential oils have been around for thousands of years, dating as far back to biblical times. In fact, essential oils have been specifically mentioned several times throughout the Bible and documented in various medical texts throughout history!

These oils weren't just around for therapeutic purposes and because they smelt good. These oils hold the secret to a powerful, ancient form of healing, back when modern day hospitals and synthetically-produced drugs were not even in existence yet. Humans back then relied on these essential oils to cure any ailments, aches, pains, colds, and illnesses they contracted, and it is how we as a species have managed to survive and thrive all this time.

Today, essential oils are still as powerful as they were back then. Many of them can be found among our common household items as moisturizers, health boosters, and even as cleaning products. In this book, you are going to explore the rich history of essential oils, why they are so powerful, what side effects they come with, how to take your health to new heights with these oils, and even how to use them in everyday personal care and around your home.

Due to this big boom in the use of essences, there are now millions of books on the market that will help you to understand what exactly these essences can do for you. In this book, I am referring to these essences as aromatic oils. This is simply to pay homage to the fact that they are not only medicinal in purpose but also therapeutic.

There are plenty of books on this subject on the market. Thanks again for choosing this one! Every effort was made to ensure it is full of as much useful information as possible. Please enjoy!

Chapter 1: An Introduction to Essential Oils and Its History

You're probably already familiar with some of the essential oils. In fact, you have probably even used them during your routine massage sessions at the spa or on your face as part of your skincare routine. What are these essential oils anyway and how did they gain popularity the way they did? Let's find out.

To better understand what essential oils encompass, we need to look a little deeper into the subject. There are two types of essential oils: volatile oils and fixed oils.

Volatile oils have a very different function and purpose to the fixed oils. Because volatile oils tend to evaporate easily, they are commonly used as skin care products since they absorb easily when applied topically. The oil's volatility is precisely what makes it so useful as an aromatherapy treatment, which is why you'll find your favorite masseuse applying a generous amount on your body whenever you have your massage session. The delicious scents that emerge from these essential oils are produced when the molecules get released into the air as vapor.

Fixed oils, on the other hand, are oils derived from either plants or animals. They are not naturally volatile, which means they do not evaporate. Some common household examples of fixed oils that you might already have in your kitchen right now include coconut oil, grape seed oil, and even olive oil that is a common oil which is now used in many cooking recipes.

As an example to illustrate the difference between fixed and volatile oils, try this little experiment. Apply a coating of coconut oil (fixed oil) onto one hand. What does your hand look like 2-3 minutes later? Probably still greasy and oily-looking. Now, in comparison, apply a coating of frankincense oil (volatile oil) to your skin for example. Take a look at your hand 2-3 minutes later, and you'll probably find no visible traces of the oil on your skin any longer because it would have evaporated and been absorbed into your skin. That's the difference between fixed and volatile essential oils. They're both still essential, just different in nature.

Where Do These Essential Oils Come From?

Most essential oils come directly from plants, including leaves, flowers, barks, roots, and even peels. These plants are then put through a steam-distillation process, where it gets cold-pressed or is extracted using the CO_2. To maintain the essence of these oils, the extraction process should not involve the use of any chemical solvents in the mix. That is how the essential oils are kept as pure as possible.

Why Do We Call Them Essential Oils?

When you think of the word *'essential'*, it often implies that this is something that is a necessity, something that you simply must have, and something that you can't do without in your life. For example, consuming fruits and vegetables are essential because our bodies need the vitamins, nutrition, and minerals which are produced by these foods to remain in optimum health.

When something is essential to the human body, it is often because our bodies cannot produce what we need on our own. Amino acids, for example, are something which is essential and what we cannot produce alone, which is why we need to eat to survive (amino acids are derived from our food source). So, by that logic, if essential oils are called *'essential* oils', does that mean we need them to survive too?

Not exactly. Our bodies can do just fine without them. Essential oils are short for *'quintessential'*, which means *"processing or embodying an essence"*. The "essence" in this case, would be the oils. Instead of calling them quintessential oils, we call them essential oils.

Quintessential (also referred to as *quinta essentia*), when translated literally, means *"the fifth element"*. Back in ancient times, it was believed that the fifth element was the highest element that could be achieved. It was also believed that when the fifth element was combined with other elements like water, air, or fire, it created an entirely new state of being.

Essential oils are considered the spirit of the plant—its very essence. This essence can help support the human body's health system in more ways than we could ever imagine. The dawn of modern medicine and drugs as a way to cure what ails us may be the norm, but in ancient times, the early humans relied on essential oils for their health before the existence of the hospitals, medicinal drugs, and equipment that we know today.

The History of Essential Oils

Essential oils have a history which can be traced as far back as the biblical age. In fact, essential oils have been mentioned several times throughout the Bible in various passages. It is easy to dismiss these traditional treatments and remedies as old wives' tales, something that isn't as effective as modern day medicine is. However, sometimes, what you find in nature can hold a cure that is more powerful and effective than any medicinal drug can ever be.

Essential oils were used as a form of ancient medicine because the early humans back then could literally find anything they needed to cure their ailments within nature. The options were vast, and the side effects were less worrying the way modern medicine is. The results even lasted much longer too. For thousands of years, these oils were very much an integral part of the people's lives. Throughout the Bible, several essential oils were mentioned in different passages. Within the Bible, these oils were referred to using terms like ointments, perfumes, aromas, fragrances, odors, and even sweet savors.

Hyssop, frankincense and myrrh, and rosemary were some of the common oils used in the Bible for the anointing and healing of the sick. In the Old Testament, it is pointed out that Moses and other important figures used essential oils when they were anointing leaders and kings. Priests were also mentioned to use these oils for healing purposes. The most infamous story in the Bible, the one which told of Jesus' birth in the manger, also points out how the three wise men came from afar to offer several gifts to the King, including frankincense and myrrh as the anointing oil. In historical times, it was frankincense oil—due to its anti-inflammatory properties—which was often rubbed on children to help minimize any swelling and provide immunity protection for them. Myrrh, on the other hand, was a natural antiseptic oil, which helped to heal tissues and balance out the body's hormone levels.

These wonderful, natural resources were how people throughout history have kept their health and well-being in optimal condition. The Ancient Egyptians also had a great love for essential oils and these were frequently used in the embalming and mummification process. Essential oils, which included juniper berry, spikenard, cedarwood, cinnamon, and myrrh, were used to help preserve the bodies, especially of Pharaohs and other royalty as they were prepped and prepared for the afterlife. When King Tut's tomb was uncovered by archeologists back in 1923, among the discoveries were alabaster jars which contained essential oils.

The ancient Egyptians were also famous for burning incense when they honored their gods because they firmly believed that the aromatic smoke emitted from the incense would go up to the heavens. Along with it, the smoke would carry all their prayers which they wanted to be answered. There were temples used for producing and blending essential oils that have been recorded throughout history in Egypt. Oil recipes could even be found written in hieroglyphics on the walls of these temples. That was how significant essential oils were at the time. Egyptian women were even famous for bathing themselves in these essential oils to help keep their skin rejuvenated. Cleopatra, one of the most famous Egyptian women in history, used oils like rose, cypress, myrrh, and neroli as part of her beauty regiment. She was considered to be one of the most beautiful women in the world.

The ancient Chinese were also firm believers in the power of essential oils as ancient medicine. Shennong's Herbal is the oldest Chinese text in existence, dating back to 2700 B.C., written by Shennong who was considered a mythical sage ruler in prehistoric China. It was reported that he actually consumed hundreds of herbs during his time to test out their medicinal value. The ancient Chinese used essential oils along with other ingredients as an advanced form of holistic healing, tapping into the power of these essential oils and their healing properties to help sustain their health for thousands of years.

Essential oils have even shown up in ancient Greek, where it is believed that Hippocrates, whom many credit as the *'Father of Western Medicine'*, documented over 200 different types of herbs during his lifetime. He believed that these plant-based medicines were the first key to saving lives and that any form of surgery should only be seen as a last resort measure.

During the 1800s, pharmaceutical companies start to emerge, many of whom are still in existence today, including Abbott and Parke-Davis. Companies like Pfizer, Johnson & Johnson, and Merck would later go on to become the mainstream drug companies that we know today. Back then, these companies were still using plant-based medicines as synthetic drugs began gaining momentum and popularity.

By the time the 20th century hit, people had stopped turning to plant-based medicines in favor of manufactured drugs instead, which offered a quicker, more convenient, and effective solution. Aromatherapy only made a comeback in the U.S. around the 1980s, as product makers started using these essential oils once more in the production of lotions, perfumes, and candles.

Essential Oils Today

As we are beginning to rediscover its benefits and uses, essential oils are gaining in popularity once again, especially in skincare products. However, there is so much more uses and benefits to these oils, which can do wonders to increase your health and vitality, as you will go on to discover within the other chapters of this book.

Chapter 1bis: The History of This Natural Alternative to Modern Medicine

The history of aromatic oils in medicinal uses is widespread and spans over the course of 15,000 years. With the extensive history of the aromatic and medicinal uses of these oils, it is not a surprise that many people are using them today. When modern medicine came into the mainstream, many people feared what they did not know about it. They considered it the works of the devil like magic people since they were seeing improvements. However, they never took the time to test the resulting effects in the long run. With essence, there are thousands of years of long-running tests that prove not only the validity of the benefits but also provide us with a basis by which to understand what we are doing and how to effectively use them for the purpose of healing our families.

Throughout history, you will find that plants are used for about everything. We use plants for food, for medicine, for harvesting and housing, as well as for clothing, and entertainment. Today, the plant provides resources for the world that includes:

- Spices
- Timber
- Paper
- Wheat
- Rice
- Tobacco
- Fruit
- Vegetables
- Clothing
- Nutrients
- Warmth
- Oxygen
- And so much more

When Gattefosse decided to take his own health into his own hands and treat himself with lavender oil after a horrendous laboratory fire, he learned that the use of this oil healed his skin. Without his documented proof of the validity of the benefits, society would consider aromatic oils more alternative than they do. However, due to his recorded and documented healing process, society has found that the use of plants is much vaster than they first believed.

Although aromatic oils have been used for centuries to help with perfumes, healing, anointing, and food, many people did not believe in the medicinal properties of these plants and oils. In fact, in the 1800s, many people were utilizing the medicinal properties of oils for their homes. A few scientists once started using essences in a laboratory-type setting where they were able to develop a method by which you could use nature to make people whole again. Once the Bubonic Plague started, many cities would burn frankincense and pine in the streets to ward off the evil that the Bubonic Plague brought. Later records showed that those cities had fewer incidents of Plague and death than other cities. After this time period, many people started to use aromatic oils to fragrant their homes, their clothes, linens, and for medicinal uses. After several thousand years, the use of aromatic plants and oils had spread its reach from Ancient Egypt, China, and India all the way to the United States.

In the Middle Ages and Renaissance periods, the religious were made to believe that using perfume was an excessive act of beautification, and it subsequently declined in use. This brought on a change to the use of aromatic oils. This is also the time period when incense was brought into the church for a blessing to God. It was believed that the foul odors that would permeate through the streets were an insult to God, so they would use incense to cleanse the air for him. When the citizens wanted to ward off the bad air, they would wear something called pomanders or incense necklace. These amulets would be dosed in the essences of the plants in order to provide an aromatic charm against any bad airs.

Due to the use of the amulets with the essences, an apothecary was opened to provide the essence for those wishing to wear a pomander. This was made ever popular when Queen Elizabeth started to create her own personal blend. In that day, what we would consider a perfumer now was called a pharmacist. This brought about a large range of medicinal uses and therapeutic uses that made their way into the homes of the commoners. The pharmacists would blend concoctions and create medicinal blends from new aromatics that were located around the continent.

This brought a mainstream use of aromatherapy to many cultures in that time period. It also brought aromatherapy to the commoner who, otherwise, would not have had access to these unbelievably expensive and rare ingredients. This led us to the 18th and 19th century when perfume became a means of seducing the opposite sex and a way for those that wore it to show their hierarchy and attractiveness to others. When bathing became a more commonplace activity and was viewed as a more important aspect to keeping germs at bay, the use of perfumes changed. It was no longer a necessary process to bath in the aromatic perfumes for their ability to cover the odor. Instead, the scents that became popular turned to soft floral-and citrus-based scents. This led us to the use of aromatics as a medicinal benefit after Gattefosse accidentally stuck his hand in a vat of Lavender oil after burning it in a fire at his lab.

Chapter 2: Why Essential Oils Are so Powerful & the Dangerous Side Effects

Did you know that a lot of today's modern medicine still includes compounds in them which are derived from plants? Looks like the ancient plant-based healing methods have not completely died out after all. Herbalists, especially, have always touted the benefits and they have been using botanicals in their healing remedies for generations. Natural healers are also a big believer in plant-based healing. Essential oils are making a comeback, especially when it's starting to become obvious just how effective they can be.

Why Essential Oils Are so Powerful

These oils are extracted directly from the plant. It is the *life force* of the plant, helping it to survive and thrive in its environment; that's what makes these oils so powerful when used correctly. It is the very essence of what helps to keep the plant alive. These oils are powerful because they can travel throughout our bodies, to cleanse and repair us from within, to address the health issues we may be experiencing at the *source,* and to help boost our immune system and keeps our bodies functioning in optimal condition.

Because these oils are so concentrated, a little goes a long way that's enough to pack a powerful punch. For example, it only takes 22 seconds for the molecules to reach your brain when you inhale an essential oil. When you apply it topically on your skin, just one drop is sometimes all it takes. Within a minute or two, it gets absorbed and travels into your bloodstream, and in only 20 minutes, every part and cell in your body will be feeling the effects of these essential oils. That's how powerful they are, more effective than any pharmaceutical cream or ointment out there.

While using essential oil for therapeutic purposes in the U.S. is still not as widespread right now, medical aromatherapy is more common in Europe. Here, you will find that it's common for a treatment plan to be accompanied with essential oils. However, although essential oils can improve and enhance your life and your health in many ways, they are not a cure-all solution. Serious diseases still require a supervised treatment plan by your doctor, and in no way should you rely on essential oils alone to cure any serious conditions you may have, especially if they are naturally life-threatening.

The Harvard School of Public Health once published an article that mentioned there were nearly 128,000 deaths per year and approximately 2 million hospitalizations because of prescription medications. This is proof that prescription drugs are a health risk, despite being designed to target the symptoms of your disease and treat them. However, although they do a good job targeting the symptoms, they rarely ever get to the *root* of the problem to cure it at the source. Pharmaceutical drugs can do wonders and have been great at curing a lot of conditions which several years ago may have seemed like a lost cause, but there was also a time before modern medicine existed when plant-based medicinal options were used to treat the various human conditions.

In 2014, the United States National Library of Medicine published a scientific review where essential oils underwent safety testing and displayed very minimal negative side effects and risks if used as properly directed. In fact, the review revealed that some essential oils had been approved for use as ingredients in food, where they were classified under Generally Recognized As Safe (GRAS) by the United States Food and Drug Administration when used within specific limits. Of course, they come with their own risk and complications, just like everything else. Labels and instructions must be read and properly adhered to, and you should be especially careful with them if you're already taking some kind of prescription drug.

How Do Essential Oils Work?

Plants are so much more than just flowers, leaves, barks, and roots. They have more to give, so much more healing benefits to them. Essential oils are as powerful as they are because of the healing properties that these plants have. Plants are survivors in their own right. It is incredible how unique these plants are, the chemicals, aromas, and unique tastes and colors they can produce, all of which help to protect them from predators, keep bacteria at bay, and even encourage other animals to come and pollinate.

By extracting these essential oils from plants, we are using their magical properties to help heal and support our own bodily functions. For example, plants like thyme and oregano have been known to naturally repel pathogenic bacteria, parasites, and viruses, which help protect these plants. In that same way, we can harness these same qualities for medicinal purposes using these traits in the form of essential oil that helps cure some ailments we may experience.

More Importantly, Is It Safe to Use These Essential Oils?

Yes, if you don't overdo it that is. Just because something is deemed "natural", it doesn't mean you can go overboard with it. Anything that is taken in excess can eventually cause some side effects, essential oils included. These oils are highly concentrated compounds, and whether you're inhaling it, applying it topically, or ingesting it because it is such a concentrated substance and it comes from plants, this means that any allergy you may have towards that plant will be magnified.

If you have asthma, for example, an overpowering or strong fragrance from these oils might trigger possible respiratory reactions. If you are allergic to any plant, in particular, applying it topically on your skin, even in the form of an oil, could potentially cause skin reactions. On top of that, if you're already taking some prescribed medication, some of the medicinal properties from certain plants could disagree with your medication, which can cause a reaction.

In this case, does that mean you should stay away from essential oils if you're allergic to them and miss out on the healing benefits they bring? Not necessarily. What you could do instead is take some of the oil, dilute it with water, and try applying a small test patch on your skin to see what happens.

Additionally, you should also check with your local physician before you begin any kind of essential oil regimen if you suffer from allergies just to be on the safe side.

If you are pregnant, you should also stay away from essential oils, or be very careful about what you use. Pregnancy is a very crucial time in a woman's life, and every precaution must be taken to ensure a safe and smooth pregnancy. As beneficial as these oils may be, some oils have some with specific risk factors involved. The best thing to do would be to conduct thorough research into the oil you're thinking of using and double-check with your physician to make sure that it's safe for you to use.

It is very important to speak to a healthcare provider before you attempt to use these essential oils on your own. Some essential oils—cade oil, costus root, nightshade, sassafras, nettle, and several others—have been banned by the International Fragrance Association because they are classified as toxic when applied or ingested. Among the possible side effects you could experience with essential oil usage include:

- Skin irritation (when essential oils have been in contact with the skin for extended periods)

- Citrus oils could potentially cause sun sensitivity when applied on the skin before sun exposure
- Lavender and tea tree oils have been found to have hormone-like effects which mimic that of estrogen
- Some oils may cause a rash or burn when applied topically, like nutmeg oil
- Eucalyptus oil has been known to cause seizures if ingested
- If used in its undiluted condition, cinnamon oil can cause contact dermatitis, nausea, vomiting, facial flushing, and even double vision
- Essential oils are not safe for pregnant women, especially in the hands of untrained individuals who have never used these oils before
- Overuse can lead to seizures and allergies

Staying Safe While Using Essential Oils

Just like you would with pharmaceutical drugs, there are safety factors that you should take into account to ensure you're using these essential oils in the safest possible way. You want to benefit from their medicinal and healing properties, not make things significantly worse for yourself.

To stay safe while using essential oils, follow the safety guidelines and factors by National Association for Holistic Aromatherapy below:

- **Check the Oil's Chemical Composition:** Some oils can cause possible skin reactions, especially the ones which are rich in phenols and aldehydes. If you are using oil that's rich in any constituent, it is always best if you dilute it with some water before applying it topically on the skin, just to be safe.

- **Observe the Quality of the Oil Being Used:** The essential oils that you use should be pure, genuine, and authentic to ensure maximum health benefits. Oils used in its unadulterated form have increased the likelihood of you experiencing an adverse reaction to it, especially when you're unfamiliar about the right way to use it. Always ensure that your oils are made of nothing but the best quality, again, to be on the safe side.

- **Careful with Your Application Method:** These are several ways an essential oil can be taken. Some can be applied topically onto the skin. Some can be inhaled. Some can be ingested, while others may be diffused. With each method comes its safety considerations. The dilution ratio and dosage ratio are two things that you need to especially take note of. You should read the instructions carefully before applying or taking it. These oils are highly concentrated; the wrong dosage will increase your chances of experiencing a negative reaction or undesired health effects.

- **The State of Your Skin:** If your skin is inflamed, damaged, irritated, or experiencing a disease or skin condition, it is a lot more sensitive and prone to experiencing dermal reactions. Therefore, applying essential oils on your skin when it is in this state, especially if undiluted, may not be the best idea. It could even be dangerous when done incorrectly, depending on the condition and the oil. Children— infants and toddlers especially—have a lot more sensitive skin, so you may want to avoid using any essential oils on them.

If you are planning to use essential oils, always do so properly, read the labels and instructions very carefully, and don't be fooled by the fact that is a *natural ingredient*. It may be natural, but you still need to use as advised to avoid any of the side effects which have been mentioned above.

Chapter 3: What Do You Need to Get Started with a Proper Aromatic Oil Routine

To start a proper Aromatic Oil routine, you will need to invest in several different products. First, let us start with the oils that you will need for a basic aromatic oil collection for any household.

For any decent aromatic oil collection, you will need to have anywhere from 10-15 oils in your arsenal. Start with some simple ones that can be used for multiple purposes.

This would include:

- Tea Tree Oil
- Lavender Oil
- Lemon Oil
- Peppermint Oil
- Cinnamon Oil
- Frankincense Oil
- Rosemary Oil
- Wild Orange Oil
- Ginger Oil

- Myrrh Oil
- Eucalyptus Oil

Each one of these oils is an aromatic ingredient that you will need to maintain your families' health and have a well-balanced aromatic oil collection.

Below are small details about each one of these oils and what benefits they provide for your family.

Eucalyptus Aromatic Oil

Scientific term: Eucalyptus globulus
Scent: camphor-like, fresh

- Cooling
- Insect repellent
- Refreshing
- Pain reliever
- Congestion aid
- Inflammatory aid
- Breathing aid

Cinnamon Leaf and Bark Aromatic Oil

Scientific name: Cinnamomum zeylanicum

Scent: cinnamon

- Insect repellent
- Appetite increaser
- Pain reducer
- Body warmer
- Uplifting the mood of all those around
- Digestive aid
- Disinfectant
- Cellulite reduction of deposits
- Fatigue is relieved
- Aphrodisiac
- Muscle tightness is relieved

Lemon Aromatic Oil

Scientific name: Citrus limonum

Scent: Lemony

- Insect bites are soothed
- Cellulite reduction of deposits
- Fatigue is improved
- Refreshing

- Injuries that bleed are stopped easily
- Purifies the body
- Uplifting the moods of others around
- Balancing the environment
- Energizing those around
- Calming the mind
- Body is cooled
- The nervous system is in balance
- Mental clarity is increased
- Memory works better

Myrrh Aromatic Oil

Scientific name: Commiphora myrrha
Scent: bitter

- Skin rejuvenating and healing
- Inflammatory relief
- Uplifting the moods of those around
- Aid in proper meditation

Tea Tree Aromatic Oil

Scientific name: Melaleuca alternifolia
Scent: Camphor like

- Skin healing and rejuvenating
- Breathing helped through the use of vapors
- Pain is lessened
- Disinfectant

Lavender Aromatic Oil

Scientific name: Lavandula officinalis
Scent: clean and fresh

- Insect repellent
- Skin healing and rejuvenating
- Digestion aid
- Uplifting the mood of those around
- Disinfectant
- Body purifying
- Breathing aid with the use of vapes
- Pain is lessened
- Stimulating in larger portions
- Stress reduction
- Calming in small portions
- Congestion is broken down
- Inflammation is reduced
- Mood swings are balanced
- Sleep is more restful
- Muscles that are tight are loosened

Peppermint Aromatic Oil

Scientific name: Mentha piperita
Scent: minty and strong

- Insect repellant
- Digestion relief
- Congestion relief
- Breathing is improved with the use of vapors
- Refreshing
- Pain is relieved
- Uplifts the moods of all those around
- Body is cooled
- Fatigue is reduced
- Stimulates the nerves
- Inflammation is relieved
- Physical strength is increased
- Aphrodisiac
- Energizing
- Appetite is improved
- Lactation from breastfeeding moms is reduced
- Mental clarity is increased
- Itchy skin relief
- Memory improved

Frankincense Aromatic Oil

Scientific name: Boswellia thurifera
Scent: camphor-like and woodsy

- Skin is healed
- Reduces wrinkles
- Inflammation is lessened
- Sleep is promoted
- Calming
- Communication is encouraged

Rosemary Aromatic Oil

Scientific name: Rosmarinus officinalis
Scent: camphor and strong

- Insect repellant
- Stimulating to the nerves
- Pain is relieved
- Muscles that are tight are relaxed
- Energizing
- Aids breathing with help from vapors
- Digestion improvement
- Mental clarity improves
- Memory is improved
- Cellulite reduced deposits

- Body is purified
- Uplifting the mood of those around
- Fatigue is lessened

Sweet Orange Aromatic Oil

Scientific name: citrus aurantium

Scent: orange and sweet

- Body is purified
- Calming
- Stress is reduced
- Body is cooled
- Sleep is restored
- Uplifted the moods of those around

Ginger Aromatic Oil

Scientific name: Zingiber officinale

Scent: Spicy

- Mental clarity is improved
- Energizing
- Pain is relieved
- Memory is improved
- Appetite is improved

- Aphrodisiac
- Uplifting the moods of those around
- Pain is relieved
- Body is warmed
- Muscles that are tight are relaxed more
- Fatigue is relieved
- Digestion is improved

Other supplies that you will need are:

Carrier Oils

- Almond
- Coconut
- Aloe Vera
- Grapeseed
- Kukui
- Jojoba
- Witch hazel
- Olive oil

Measuring the Carrier Oils

Each carrier oil is added in a specific measurement:
The carrier oil is applied in ounces:

½ ounces

.5% = 1-2 drops

1% = 3 drops

2.5% = 7-8 drops

3% = 9 drops

5% = 15 drops

10% = 30 drops

1 ounce

.5% = 3 drops

1% = 6 drops

2.5% = 15 drops

3% = 18 drops

5% = 30 drops

10% = 60 drops

2 ounces

.5% = 6 drops

1% = 12 drops

2.5% = 30 drops

3% = 36 drops

5% = 60 drops

10% = 120 drops

4 ounces

.5% = 12 drops

1% = 24 drops

2.5% = 60 drops

3% = 72 drops

5% = 120 drops

10% = 240 drops

You will also need ways to blend the oils. This would involve glass bowls, drams for storage, spray bottles, and even containers for lotions, salves, and roller application.

Once you have collected all of these supplies, you will need to store your oils in a cabinet that is kept away from heat and light. This will ensure that the oils stay healthy for the longest time possible.

Knowing the profiles of Aromatic Oils

Antiseptic Aromatic Oils

- Bergamot Aromatic Oil
- Clary Sage Aromatic Oil
- Cedarwood Aromatic Oil
- Peppermint Aromatic Oil
- Thyme Aromatic Oil
- Clove Aromatic Oil
- Chamomile Aromatic Oil
- Rosemary Aromatic Oil

- Eucalyptus Aromatic Oil
- Jasmine Aromatic Oil
- Cinnamon Aromatic Oil
- Juniper Aromatic Oil
- Grapefruit Aromatic Oil
- Lemon Aromatic Oil
- Ylang-Ylang Aromatic Oil
- Orange Aromatic Oil
- Myrrh Aromatic Oil
- Sandalwood Aromatic Oil
- Patchouli Aromatic Oil
- Lavender Aromatic Oil

Antibiotic Aromatic Oils

- Bergamot Aromatic Oil
- Clove Aromatic Oil
- Cinnamon Aromatic Oil
- Lavender Aromatic Oil
- Lemon Aromatic Oil
- Eucalyptus Aromatic Oil
- Thyme Aromatic Oil
- Tea Tree Aromatic Oil
- Geranium Aromatic Oil
- Patchouli Aromatic Oil

Antifungal Aromatic Oil

- Tea Tree Aromatic Oil
- Cedarwood Aromatic Oil
- Myrrh Aromatic Oil
- Patchouli Aromatic Oil
- Clove Aromatic Oil
- Eucalyptus Aromatic Oil

Antiviral Aromatic Oil

- Thyme Aromatic Oil
- Eucalyptus Aromatic Oil
- Melissa Aromatic Oil
- Clove Aromatic Oil
- Cinnamon Aromatic Oil
- Tea Tree Aromatic Oil

Anti-infectious Aromatic Oil

- Lavender Aromatic Oil
- Peppermint Aromatic Oil
- Sandalwood Aromatic Oil
- Chamomile Aromatic Oil
- Patchouli Aromatic Oil

- Thyme Aromatic Oil
- Eucalyptus Aromatic Oil
- Lemon Aromatic Oil
- Clary Sage Aromatic Oil
- Palmarosa Aromatic Oil

To measure your Essences properly

Below is a simplified chart:

20 drops=1 ml
1 tsp/100 drops =5 ml
200 drops/1/3 ounce/ 2 tsp =10 ml
300 drops/1/2 ounce/1 tbsp =15 ml
600 drops/1 ounce/ 2 tbsp =30 ml
1200 drops/2 ounces/4 tbsp/ =60 ml
2400 drops/4 ounces/ 8 tbsp/½ cup=120 ml
3600 drops/8 ounces/16 tbsp/1 cup=240 ml

Now you will need to know the dilution ratio per drops, tsp, tbsp, ounces, and cups that are safe.

Chapter 4: Common Techniques and Tools to Use for Your Aromatic Oils

Incorporating a daily practice into your life

After you have collected all the supplies that you will need, you should begin to practice making blends and learning all you can about how to use aromatic oils for your express purposes.

You can do this by experimenting with aromas in your diffuser or on a handkerchief. Another way to experiment is to try to solve household problems with a few blends that will not harm anyone in the home. A few of the blends listed in this book will help you to gain a bit of insight into all the uses that aromatic oils can provide for your family and home environment.

A few ways to incorporate the use of aromatic oils into your life is to use these oils in your hair care products.

By adding together a few oils into a hair tonic blend and eliminating the shampoos that are loaded with toxic chemicals that weigh your hair down, you can begin to have a healthier hair that is lush and full. A few ingredients that can be added to a hair tonic are:

- Coco butter
- Rosemary
- Lemongrass
- Tea Tree
- Lavender
- Orange
- Grapefruit
- Cedarwood
- Sage
- Peppermint
- Eucalyptus
- Sandalwood
- Ginger
- Hazelnut
- Lime
- Ylang-Ylang
- Jojoba
- Sweet Bay
- Geranium
- Thyme
- Chamomile

- Bois de rose
- Petitgrain

Another way that you can incorporate aromatic oils into your daily practice is to create a facial that will replenish your skin's youth and complexion. One way to do this is to create a lotion that will replenish all the nutrients that you lose in your skin when you use makeup.

Some of the available oils for this type of blend are:

- Chamomile
- Hazelnut
- Lavender
- Sandalwood
- Bois de rose
- Rosemary
- Geranium
- Palmarosa
- Fennel
- Patchouli
- Frankincense
- Rose
- Jasmine
- Benzoin
- Ylang-Ylang

- Cypress
- Orange
- Lemon
- Grapeseed
- Juniper Berries
- Borage
- Myrrh
- Kukui nut
- Lime
- Avocado
- Flaxseed
- Jojoba
- Sesame
- Evening Primrose
- Tea Tree

To incorporate aromatic oils into your daily routine in a different way would be by adding oils to a bath or a diffuser for aromatic therapy. There are a large variety of oils that can be used for these types of applications. When adding oils to your bath, you need to verify that you are not allergic to them first. Afterward, you can begin to have some very aromatic baths every day.

The best oils for this application would be:

- Cajeput
- Peppermint
- Rosemary
- Lavender
- Myrtle
- Lemon
- Anise
- Eucalyptus
- Spruce
- Chamomile
- Grapefruit
- Petitgrain
- Marjoram
- Benzoin
- Fennel
- Orange
- Allspice
- Mandarin
- Palmarose
- Bergamot
- Clary Sage
- Sandalwood
- Ylang Ylang
- Patchouli
- Bois de rose

- Sweet Basil
- Nutmeg
- Lemongrass
- Geranium
- Melissa
- Juniper Berries
- Spearmint
- Cypress

Now, if you are trying to incorporate aromatic oils into your household cleaning routine, then there are a few oils that will make that easier to do. Several of these oils can be blended or you can simply use them on their own.

- Tea Tree
- Lemon
- Grapefruit
- Orange
- Rosemary
- Lavender
- Peppermint
- Eucalyptus
- Cinnamon
- Thyme

- Pine

This is just a few examples of how you can incorporate aromatic oils into your daily activities. As an avid enthusiast for aromatic oils, I know how difficult it can be to learn every aspect about aromatic oils, so take your time and explore all the oils that interest you. You will see, as I did, that once you get started, you will find some oils that you never leave home without, and then there are some that you barely ever use.

In the rest of this book, I have included several recipes that will help you to have a starting point for building your aromatic oil recipes. I hope that you find them just as useful as I have.

Chapter 5: Taking Your Health to New Heights with Essential Oils

Although modern medicine has helped in many ways, there is no denying that these synthetically-produced drugs still come with possible dangerous side effects. Every pro has its con, just like essential oils do too. In 2006, there was an independent review which was funded by the Nutrition Institute of America entitled *Death by Medicine* wherein researchers discovered that one of America's leading causes of death was a result of conventional medicine.

With essential oils, on the other hand, the side effects are not as drastic (unless you have an allergic reaction to the substance). Because essential oils have a chemical structure, it makes it easier for them to metabolize in the cells, the way that other nutrients would—especially the oils that are naturally volatile. Unlike the synthetic drugs, essential oils get absorbed quickly in the body and this makes it a much safer, natural alternative.

Indeed, essential oils are a powerful form of plant-based medicine. They are part of a plant's life force, circulating throughout the plant, carrying the nutrition into the plant's cells, and eliminating any waste. In a plant, essential oils have a healing intent, restoring balance, and helping the plant thrive. In the same way, the purest form of essential oils can help to restore balance, health, and harmony into our bodies from within. This makes them a powerful form of plant-based medicine which, when used correctly, can help take the health of your family to new heights.

According to research, people who consistently use essential oils as part of their health upkeep have been found to have a much higher tolerance and resistance towards illnesses: colds, flu, and other diseases that often tend to plague the average person. It was also discovered that individuals who frequently used essential oils recovered much faster than those who didn't when they fell ill.

Using Essential Oils to Improve Your Family's Health

If there is an option to maintain good health naturally, you should always choose that option. Natural remedies are better than synthetically-produced drugs on any given day, especially essential oils because they are derived from natural resources (plants). Various oils come with different benefits, and here we will take a look at how you can use some of these oils to improve your health and that of your family.

Basil Oil - Sometimes referred to as "sweet basil oil", it is commonly used to counter venoms from a snake or insect bites. It is also used in both Chinese and Ayurvedic medicine to treat colds, muscle aches, flu, fever, and earaches. A 2014 review published indicated that this oil has been effectively used as a traditional medicinal plant to help cure kidney malfunctions, headaches, coughing, constipation, warts, worms, and more. The key benefits of this oil are as follows: the potential to reduce inflammation, combats free-radical damage, helps relieve congestion, stimulates the nervous system, has antibacterial properties, and aids in ear infections. Do not use during pregnancy or if you have epilepsy.

Bergamot Oil - This oil is native to Southeast Asia. A study conducted in 2011 found some of the key benefits of this oil which include helping with depression or anxiety, reducing stress, minimizing pulse rate and blood pressure, soothing skin irritations, joint and muscle pain relief, and even acts as a natural deodorant.

Cardamom Oil - This oil was highly valued in ancient Rome and Greece. There have been notable mentions of this oil in medical documents dating as far back as the 16th century B.C. Egyptians used this oil for medicinal purposes and the embalming process. Key benefits of this oil include treating colic, colds, diarrhea, nausea, gas, kidney, and reproductive issues, soothing the throat, easing mental fatigues, improving respiratory conditions, and may even alleviate cramps and muscle spasms.

Citronella Oil - In Chinese medicine, this oil is used to treat aches and pains in the joints and muscles. It has also been used for centuries in China, Sri Lanka, and Indonesia to help minimize rashes, inflammation, infections, and even to repel insects. Key benefits of this oil include helping to promote relaxation, soothing muscle pain, fighting free-radical damage, reducing inflammation, repelling insects, and helping to decrease respiratory infections.

Clary Sage Oil – This oil is used in Chinese medicine to help strengthen the kidneys, female reproductive organs, and adrenal glands. In the Middle Ages, this oil was known as 'Oculus Christi', which means 'Eyes of Christ'. This oil is considered among the top essential oils for balancing hormones in women and is highly beneficial for dealing with menstrual cramps, hormonal imbalances, and hot flashes. Other key benefits of this oil include boosting eye, skin, and hair health, may provide some relief for asthma symptoms, improving moods, and helping to reduce stress.

Cypress Oil - Key benefits of this oil include helping to boost moods, possibly improve carpal tunnel syndrome, acting as a natural deodorant, stress relief, having antibacterial and antiseptic properties, may minimize varicose veins, and helping with anxiety.

Coconut Oil – This is another oil which is a common household item today. The key benefits include helping to protect skin and hair, improving mental clarity, minimizing cellulite, and keeping bacteria and fungi at bay.

Eucalyptus Oil – This is effective in helping to alleviate pain, swelling, and inflammation. Other key benefits of this oil include serving as a remedy for skin irritations and insect bites, reducing muscle pain, helping to fight infection, boosting mental clarity, relieving respiratory conditions, and may even reduce fever.

Frankincense Oil – This oil is often referred to as the *'King of Oils'* because it was mentioned several times throughout the Bible, and is famous for its healing properties. In 2011, a study conducted found that frankincense oil helped to alleviate the symptoms of gingivitis because of the anti-inflammatory properties it possesses. Other key benefits of this oil include minimizing the signs of aging, easing digestion, encouraging healthy hormone levels, supporting the body's immunity to prevent illness, having anti-tumor properties, and heightening spiritual awareness.

Jasmine Oil – This is a popular natural remedy to help improve moods, overcome stress, and balancing hormone levels. This is a natural treatment for anxiety, depression, insomnia, and low libido. Other key benefits of this oil include helping to enhance alertness and improve energy levels, promoting restful sleep, aiding in pain relief, and relieving symptoms of anxiety. This oil may even serve as an aphrodisiac.

Jojoba Oil - Another infamous oil, its key health benefits include acting as a skin moisturizer, boosting skin and hair health, stimulating collagen synthesis, helping to speed up wound closures, and helping to fight bacteria and fungi.

Lavender Oil - According to ancient medical texts, this oil has been used for both religious and medicinal purposes for over 2,500 years. It is also among the most commonly used essential oils in the world today. Thanks to its versatile and relaxing properties, lavender oil helps to promote peaceful sleep and ease feelings of tension. Other key benefits of this oil include helping with skin conditions like eczema and psoriasis, relieving headaches, promoting balanced blood sugar, helping to lower blood pressure, improving skin conditions, reducing acne, and acting as a first aid treatment for burns and wounds.

Lemongrass Oil – This oil is used in aromatherapy treatments to help alleviate muscle pain, fight bacteria, reduce body aches, and aid digestion. Other key benefits of this oil include acting as an aid to help reduce fever, boosting energy levels, reducing stomach aches, having antifungal and anti-yeast properties, and even as a relief for aches in the ligaments and tendons.

Melaleuca Oil - Better known as tea tree oil, healers used this back in the day to cure serious illnesses. This oil has also been documented for over 70 years in various medical studies as a way of killing many strains of fungi, viruses, and bacteria. Other key benefits of this oil include bad breath remedy, preventing and killing head lice, acting as a treatment for chickenpox, serving as a natural deodorant, acne treatment, relieving cold sores, and even easing earaches.

Rosemary Oil - A powerful natural health booster, this oil has some of the key benefits which include relief in muscular aches and pains, promoting hormone balance, improving alertness, regenerating nerve tissue, helping to thicken hair, and may even help to improve cognitive abilities.

Rosehip Oil - This oil is famous for its powerful antioxidants, vitamins, and essential fatty acids. Key benefits of this oil include stimulating collagen production, acting as a skin and hair moisturizer, protection from the UV rays of the sun and sun damage, having anti-aging properties, and even minimizing the appearance of fine lines and wrinkles.

Safety Guidelines and Recommendations When Using Essential Oils

A little goes a long way when it comes to using essential oils. It is important to use these oils as instructed to experience the maximum health benefits that come with regular application. If you are just starting on these oils, it is advisable that you attempt a test patch on your skin with just one or two drops to see if you experience any reaction or side effects before you continue.

While many oils can be applied undiluted or without a carrier oil, it is important that you double-check to make sure it's safe for you to do so before you proceed. If you have any doubts at all, the best thing to do would be to dilute it. If you experience any irritation in spite of diluting the oil, you should stop using it immediately. Do not attempt to use essential oils in either the eyes or ear canals.

Bear in mind that not all oils are safe for consumption. Always check the warning labels and usage guidelines before you attempt to consume or ingest any kind of essential oil. Look for indicators which show that the oil can be taken as a dietary supplement and that the oil is organic to keep its form as pure as possible. Do not ingest or use essential oils if you are pregnant. If you are consuming essential oils with other food or liquid, always put one drop first to test before attempting to go full out. It is important to note that a lot of essential oils are not meant to be taken on an empty stomach.

Make it a point to check with your healthcare provider before attempting any new regiment using these essential oils, especially if you are currently taking prescription medication, to avoid any adverse side effects. For infants, toddlers, and children, seek out the advice of the healthcare professional before attempting any essential oil treatment on them.

Chapter 6: How You Can Master Essential Oils for Home and Healthcare Needs

The craft of mastering essential oils is simple. Many people concern themselves with worry about what they are applying to their bodies. However, with essential oils, you no longer have to worry about what you are putting into your body, as long as you effectively use them. Medicines provided by medical professionals and pharmaceutical companies can be dangerous and create more ailments and disease within your body. If you have ever been to the doctor to get medicine for a disease or ailment, I am sure you have been prescribed one medication to help with one condition and another to help with the side effects of the medication prescribed. This simply means that although the doctor is supporting your use of this medication, there are side effects that will create more disease and sickness, thus requiring you to take more medication. With essential oils, this is not necessary.

Simply identify the problem that you are dealing with and then develop an essential oil blend that will help with that problem—ensuring beforehand that you are not allergic to any of the oils within the blend. If you are not allergic, then the essential oil blend will help you without requiring another medication to counteract the side effects of the oil since there will be none.

To master your own health with essential oils, you simply need to learn as much as you can about yourself and the oils that you are using. Starting with a simple set of oils is the best route to take for mastering essential oils. Learn all you can about that simple set. Once you are able to use them efficiently without consulting your manuals of books, then you can move on to new essential oils to learn how they work.

I recommend most people to start with:

Lavender = Lavandula angustifolia
Tea Tree = Melaleuca alternifolia
Sweet Orange = Citrus sinensis, citrus aurantium, sinensis
Lemon = Citrus limon
Peppermint = Mentha x Piperita

Eucalyptus = Eucalyptus globulus, E. radiata, or E. smithii

These can be purchased from any reputable essential oil company. To ensure that you have purchased your oils from a reputable company, you need to verify that they have been run through an extensive amount of testing to ensure purity and organic harvesting and growing methods.

A pure essential oil is one that is grown and cultivated from a botanical source that is specific and is not altered or modified in any way. To identify an essential oil that is of poor quality, you will need to examine the price point at which they are trying to sell them. If the price they are asking is much lower than other companies, then they are most likely not authentic. If the oils in the store are all the same price, then the same thing applies.

Next, you need to be familiar with the rarity of the oils that you are purchasing. For instance, Jasmine, Sandalwood, Rose, and Melissa are usually sold in smaller quantities due to the cost of extracting them. A ½-ounce dram of Rose oil is sold for $195 to $200—so if they are asking a price that is not in this price range, then they are not a pure, authentic, properly distilled or sourced Rose oil.

There are several purity tests that can be run on your essential oils.

Use a plain piece of white paper for watercolor. Blot a drop of oil on the paper. If the oil is not colored, then it should disappear after 48 hours without leaving a trace or aroma that has lingered. However, the more viscous the oil, the longer this test will take for evaporating with no trace.

Another test is the one where you put one drop into a glass container with water. If it discolors the water or turns milky, then it is altered with an emulsifier to hold the oil and dilution substance together.

Comparing your viscosity by dropping the essential oil between two fingers and rubbing them and then using the other hand to drop a carrier oil in the same manner and testing it, you will be able to test the viscosity of the oils. The essential oil should not have an oily texture as the carrier oil does. This can only be tested with no viscous oils.

By performing these tests, you will be able to master choosing the right essential oils for your herbal alternative medicine practice.

How Should You Use Essential Oils Safely?

Essential oils are a chemical compound. So, knowing how to use them properly. It is essential that essential oils are used in a safe and proper manner so that they do not harm you in any way or create a risk to yourself or others. Adverse effects can happen with anything, however by knowing what you are working with and the person that is using the oils you can eliminate these adverse effects in advance. There are several factors that influence the safety of an essential oil. These include:

- The method by which you are applying them.
- The dosage or dilution that is being applied.
- The quality of the essential oil that you are utilizing.
- The chemical composition that makes up the oil.
- And the integrity of the epidermis that it is being applied to.

Once you have applied these safety concerns, then you can begin to use the essential oils properly. By applying essential oils to your temples, behind the ear, on the back of the neck, forehead, wrists, the bottom of the feet, and down your back, hands or on your stomach and any muscle that pains you can begin to alleviate most to all ailments in your body.

To relieve a headache, you would apply the essential oil to your:

- Temples
- Forehead
- Behind the ears

For relieving a stomach problem, you would apply the oils to:

- The stomach or abdomen region

To relieve a fever, you would apply the oils to:

- The forehead
- Behind the neck
- On the temples
- Behind the ears
- Under the feet

To relieve sore muscles, you would apply the oil to:

- The muscle that is bothering you

To relieve sleeping problems, you would apply the oil to:

- Under the feet
- On the neck
- Behind your ears

To help someone feel calmer throughout the day, you would apply the oils to:

- The wrist
- Behind the ears
- The temples

For situations that require an inhalation method, using an inhaler is the best result or a diffuser.

To relieve a cough or chest congestion, you would apply the oils to:

- The chest
- Under the nose
- Or in a diffuser

For flue or influenzas, you would apply the oil to:

- The spine of the person who is sick
- On the back of the neck
- On the lungs area
- Under the nose
- In the diffuser

These are just a few of the locations that you would apply essential oils for proper usage. There are several methods to use essential oils and by simply knowing what you are trying to accomplish you will be able to determine the application method.

Proper Blending Techniques and Tips

To blend an essential oil with another one, you will first need to determine which oils you are blending. Many oils will go together and create a proper synergistic blend. However, your nose will be able to determine the appropriate blend for you. Decide which oils you are wishing to blend together. By following recipes, you can utilize a preexisting recipe however this may not suit your olfactory senses. You may find one oil in the blend to strong or not attractive to you. This is ok you can alter the blend recipe to suit your needs. Simply pick out the oils that you wish to use. Then, remove the lids, making sure that you know which lids, which are for replacing them properly later on. Then, holding the oils in your hand side by side, waft the oils past your nose as you breathe in. If the aroma is wrong, then find the one that bothers you and change it to one that works for you.

Once you have found the oils that you are going to use in your blend, you will need to determine which dilution ratio you will need to use. Each oil is rated at a specific dilution ratio. This can be anywhere from 0.3% to 10% dilution ratio. This means that for every number of drops there is a ratio of dilution.

To measure a proper amount of essential oils, you will need to know the proper drops measurements in ration to mL as well as tsp., tbsp., ounces, and cups.

Below is a simplified chart:

1 mL = 20 drops

5 mL = 100 drops/1 tsp

10 mL = 200 drops/2 tsp/1/3 ounce

15 mL = 300 drops/1 tbsp./1/2 ounce

30 mL = 600 drops/2 tbsp./1 ounce

60 mL = 1200 drops/4 tbsp./2 ounces

120 mL = 2400 drops/8 tbsp./4 ounces/ ½ cup

240 mL=3600 drops/16 tbsp./ 8 ounces/ 1 cup

Now, you will need to know the dilution ratios per drop, tsp, tbsp., ounce, and cup that are safe.

The carrier oil is applied in ounces:

½ ounces

.5% for every 1-2 drops

1% for every 3 drops

2.5% for every 7-8 drops

3% for every 9 drops

5% for every 15 drops

10% for every 30 drops

1 ounce

.5% for every 3 drops

1% for every 6 drops

2.5% for every 15 drops

3% for every 18 drops

5% for every 30 drops

10% for every 60 drops

2 ounces

.5% for every 6 drops

1% for every 12 drops

2.5% for every 30 drops

3% for every 36 drops

5% for every 60 drops

10% for every 120 drops

4 ounces

.5% for every 12 drops

1% for every 24 drops

2.5% for every 60 drops

3% for every 72 drops

5% for every 120 drops

10% for every 240 drops

Next, you will need to know the blending factor by which each essential oil is prepared by. This is a rate of 1-10 blending factor.

1 means that it is an aroma that is powerful, and you need less to blend.

10 means that it is much more volatile and has a lighter aromatic smell. This would mean that you need more for your blend.

Anything in between 1-10 is determined by the aromatic strength and potency. This can be determined by a simple chart for blending factors or by rating them based on your olfactory senses.

Once you have your blending factor you can begin to determine the number of drops that you will need for each blend. Start each blend with a total drops number of 30. Then, determine how many drops each oil will contribute by using the formula that is shown below.

For instance,
Lavender has a blending factor of 7
Sweet Marjoram has a blending factor of 3
German Chamomile has a blending factor of 1
Helichrysum has a blending factor of 5

When you add these together you get a total blending factor of 16. Now, divide this total blending factor for each by the total blending factor number.

This equation looks something like this:

7/16= .4375

5/16= .3125

1/16= .0625

3/16= .1875

You would then have the percentage by which you will divide these oils into a recipe with only using 30 drops for the whole recipe.

Lavender was a 7-blending factor with a .4375/30 which equals 13 drops.

Helichrysum was a 5-blending factor with a .3125/30 which equals 9 drops.

German chamomile was a 2-blending factor with a .0625/30 which equals 2 drops.

Sweet Marjoram was a 3-blending factor with a .1875/30 which equals 6 drops.

This should give you a basic idea of how to determine the blends that you wish to create.

Next, you will need to understand the proper way to blend an essential oil blend. The technique is pretty simple. First, once you have determined how many drops you will use form each oil, you will need to place those drops in order of the highest number of drops to the lowest number of drops, within a glass bottle or container that can be rolled between your palms. Once you have placed all your drops into the container, cap it, and then roll it between your palms. Then, place the container between your first finger and thumb and flip the bottle upside down, then right side up. This helps to blend the oils without a vigorous and aggressive force. This will not create negative energy around the blend. One key thing to remember is that while you are dripping the oils into the bottle stop after every oil that you drip in and swirl the bottle to use centripetal force to bring the oil to the bottom of the bottle. This ensures that the oils are at the bottom and not sitting on the sides. Blending your oils should be done for a maximum of 3 minutes. This will ensure a proper blend of the oils within the bottle. Always blend oils in a glass container.

Creating Your Own Blends

To create a blend, you will need to use your own olfactory senses to determine what you like together and what you do not like together. The best way to do this is by placing the oils side by side and sifting the oils back and forth across your nose and if they are a pleasant aroma to you then they are a great blend to use.

Purchasing the Best Essential Oils for Your Needs

Essential oils can be sold by many companies but there are a few that are not reputable. I have included a list of companies that have been tested and proven authentic, pure, and non-altered.

- Essential Aura Aromatherapy – www.essentialaura.com or www.organicfair.com

- Florihana – www.florihana.com

- Un9iversal Companies – www.universalcompanies.com

- Fragrant Earth – www.fragrant-earth.com

- Mountain Rose Herb – www.mountainroseherb.com

- Plant Therapy – www.planttherapy.com

Properly Storing Your Essential Oils

To safely store your essential oils, you will need to have your blends in a brown or amber glass bottle. They can last, depending on the type of oil it is, for 6 to 12 months after opened and blended. To store them properly they need to be stored in cool dry locations, that is away from sunlight and heat. Many companies will have an option for proper storage that you can purchase. This can be anything from a box that is able to store up to 64 oils as well as a portfolio type storage solution.

To ensure that you are storing your oils properly, make sure the area you use follows these rules:

- Cool
- Dry
- No sunlight
- No dampness
- No heat

Chapter 7: How to Effectively Use Essential Oils

Before you dive into the world of essential oils, you should know some of the vital information about these products to ensure that you're getting the most out of it for your health.

Getting to Know Essential Oils: How They Are Made

As we already know, essential oils are mainly derived from plants, serving very distinct purposes in nature. Each oil is designed to help the host plant survive and thrive in the environment by helping to ward off attacking organisms which may threaten the survival of the plan. The oils generated by the plant help to keep away from insects and pests which may consume or destroy the plant at bay, while at the same time helping these plants to emit the pleasant aromas which attract other insects to pollinate.

These oils are carefully extracted from the plant, and the methods of extraction would depend on the type of plant in question. It would also depend on the availability of the equipment because each oil must be carefully extracted to ensure that it stays true to its purest form. The most basic methods of extraction here include steam distillation, extraction, and expression, with steam distillation being the most commonly used method today. The steam distillation method was invented sometime in the 10th century by an Arabian physician named Avicenna, who was credited for this invention.

Using this steam distillation method, essential oils are produced and made when the plant is exposed to the steam, and the heat from the steam is what causes the essential oils to evaporate. The hot vapors are then subsequently cooled, and this causes condensation of both the oil and the vapor. Since oil and water do not mix, this makes separating the two substances a much easier process.

The plants carrying these essential oils need to be farmed in the right manner as well. The soil and the terrain where the plants are grown needs to be just the right mix to produce oils in its purest form and with the highest quality. Only knowledgeable farmers should handle the farming of these plants because they are familiar with just how much time the plant needs to reach full maturity. They also know that it is important for these plants not be exposed to any harsh pesticides or chemicals because this will affect the chemistry of the plant, which will then affect the therapeutic quality of the essential oils within the plant.

The difference in the soil, terrain, climate, and the method of harvesting all make a difference to the quality of the oils being produced. Lavender, for example, is a Mediterranean plant and it thrives best when grown in subtropical regions. Wild Alaskan blueberries have at least five times more antioxidant properties than the blueberries which are available in North America. It is best that the essential oil plants are allowed to thrive and grow in the climates and environments where they are meant as this will allow them to reach full maturity in the nutrient-rich soil they need.

Getting to Know Essential Oils: Talking About Quality

There is absolutely a difference when it comes to the quality of oils. You should never be fooled by an essential oil product just because the label on it states that it is "100% pure and natural". This doesn't necessarily mean you are getting the best quality; it could be just a label that has been slapped on for marketing purposes.

Pure, 100% unadulterated essential oils are far more difficult to come by than you would imagine. When a product is difficult to come by, that can only mean one thing: when you get your hands on it, it is going to be expensive. Did you know that to simply produce one bottle of 15ml lavender oil, it could take up to 27 square feet of lavender plants? Just to produce that one small quantity! It could take 75 lemons just to make a 15ml bottle of lemon oil, and 60 roses to make just one drop of rose oil. This is the reason why pure—*really pure*—essential oils can be such a costly affair.

High-quality essential oils *must be free* from chemicals, no exception. They must also be *very carefully* extracted to ensure that these oils are kept in their natural state. Once the oils have been extracted, they should be kept bottled in dark, glass containers to help protect them from sunlight and oxidation.

Not all essential oils are going to be of equal quality. If not properly extracted, stored, and handled, many of these oils just end up becoming worthless because you're not reaping the full benefits that you should be. Some oils could even be potentially toxic if there are too many synthetic chemicals and other additives that have been added to the mix.

The lowest quality of essential oils available is the synthetic and altered form of oils which are created in laboratories. These man-made properties are considered the lowest quality because they simply do not have the same type of healing properties the way essential oils should have. Here are the most common types of essential oil qualities:

- Essential oils that are therapeutic grade are oils which have been steam-distilled and unadulterated and could contain beneficial compounds. However, it would depend on the company that's producing them. The quality is not a guarantee here either because there is no way of guaranteeing that no chemical fertilizers or pesticides have been sprayed on the plant. Although these oils are generally considered the safest, it does not necessarily mean that they are as their quality is difficult to authenticate.

- Oils which are "100% natural" or "100% pure" are not necessarily the best quality either. These are among the most commonly available oils. That's what the label may say, but don't be fooled because these oils are overly processed too, which means that at the end of the day, their healing properties are not as effective. Some may even lose their healing properties altogether. This also in no way guarantees that no additional ingredients and compounds have been added to these oils. In the U.S., just 5% of the essential oils in a bottle is enough for you to label the bottle as "pure essential oil".

- The highest grade of essential oils with the greatest healing properties are the ones which are certified organic. There is definitely a distinctive difference between these oils and the ones mentioned above. You will be able to differentiate the quality of these oils through taste, smell, and feel. These are also the most expensive type of oils on the market because the supply is very limited and difficult to come by.

How to Assess Your Essential Oils' Quality

If you want to test out the quality and potency of the essential oil you have, here are several ways that you could do so:

- **Read the Labels** - If you know the Latin names of your oils, that would certainly be an advantage. Plants can have similar or common names but come in different varieties which can produce different results. When you purchase your oils, always make it a point to read the label and check if the correct botanical name has been printed on it.

- **Smell It** - The smell of the oil would be a good indicator of its quality. The more potent your oil smells, the more powerful and pure the oil is. Give it a good sniff before you make that purchase.

- **Look at the Price Tag -** Premium, high-quality oils tend to come with a much heftier price tag. You are paying for quality of the oil, and because they are harder to come by, they will generally be more expensive. If the price tag is significantly cheaper, the oil you're purchasing might not be the highest quality.

- **Reputation Matters -** Another key point to remember to ensure that you're only purchasing high-quality essential oils is to buy them from reputable companies. Reputable companies have a much higher standard which they go by, and you can usually trust the information printed on the product label.

Practical Tips to Use Your Essential Oils

Essential oils can emit powerful odors which can be both mentally and emotionally stimulating. Some scents have a way of relaxing and calming you just by getting a good whiff of it. Besides applying it directly on your skin as a moisturizer, here are some practical tips to using your essential oils for you to get the most out of every use:

- Directly inhale the scent by opening the bottle of essential oil and breathing in its powerful aroma. If inhaling directly might be too much for you, place a drop or two of the desired oil on your hands, rub them together and cup your hands around your nose, closing your eyes are you breathe in the scent.

- Essential oils can also be used with a diffuser, allowing the oil to evaporate into its surroundings and filling your home with a deliciously fragrant scent. Types of diffusers include atomizing, evaporation, vaporization, and heat diffusers.

- Apply a couple of drops of essential oil into your bathwater and soak in the tub for several minutes, allowing the oil to soak into your skin for a relaxing and calming bath session.

- One of the most popular ways of utilizing essential oils is during your regular massage sessions.

* **Do not attempt to ingest essential oils without first speaking to your healthcare practitioner about it.**

Chapter 8: Using Essential Oils around the Home & For Personal Care

Let's face it, we're all worried about getting more and more harmful chemicals into our body. With the dangers of phthalates found mainly in commercial air fresheners, detergents having a harmful effect on the environment, and plastic particles going into the sea, people are finding more natural ways of getting what they want without harming their body or the environment.

Essential oils are among the all-natural items making way into the households of people in America and around the world as natural solutions of cleaning, disinfecting, purifying, and scenting.

Here are the many ways essential oils can be used for housekeeping and personal care:

Home Care

- **Disinfect Your Counters**

Plenty of essential oils have antiviral, antibacterial, and antifungal elements making them well-suited to be used as simple, gentle homemade cleaning products. Making your own essential oil disinfectant not only protects you from breathing and spreading harmful chemicals but also saves you from purchasing overpriced and over-processed commercial cleaners and disinfectants.

You can create your own counter disinfectant by adding 2-3 drops of lavender, lemon, sweet orange, and even tea tree essential oil into diluted liquid castile soap. Mix all this into a small spray bottle. Once you are done with cooking, spray this concoction onto your counters so you'll have squeaky clean counters. This mixture works well on non-porous surfaces.

- **Clean Your Toilet**

The mixture you made for your countertop cleaning can also be used to keep your toilet spick and span and smelling nice. You can make your own toilet tabs by mixing 2-3 drops of lemon, sweet orange, lavender, and tea tree oil into a bowl with 1 tablespoon of baking soda. Spray this mixture lightly with water, and using silicone molds, ice cube trays, or mini muffin trays, press the baking soda essential oil mixture into the molds. Let these dry overnight, then remove them from their molds and store them in an airtight jar. Before you shower each day, toss one of these tabs into the toilet and flush it out after you are done with your shower. This keeps your toilet fresh and clean between deep cleaning sessions.

- **Boost Up the Scent of Your Laundry**

We all love the smell of freshly washed clothes, however, some detergents do not always give that fresh after-wash scent. If you want to enhance the scent of your laundry, you can definitely use essential oils to give your fabrics that clean, natural smell. All you need to do is add a few drops of your favorite scent of essential oil into your existing detergent. Among the popular favorites for fabric scent is lavender, lemon, peppermint, and ylang-ylang.

You can also add 2-3 drops of essential oil to a wool dryer ball and drop it into your dryer. Using essential oils is a hypoallergenic alternative which is not only great for your nose but also keeps your clothes soft and smelling amazing all the time.

- **Clean Your Carpets**

When you have carpets, you need to give them extra care and attention because they get dirty fast and that also means they tend to smell musty too. Having a DIY cleanser not only makes your carpets clean and smell fresh longer but also makes it affordable to have carpets. Baking soda and essential oils are a great combination as they provide the basis of many cleansers, cleaners, and sprays. Baking soda is ideal for removing food and pet odors, whereas essential oils leave your carpet fresh, clean, and smelling brand new.

For your weekly carpet cleaning, you can start off by vacuuming your carpets to pick up the dirt, fur, and dust. Next, mix 2 cups of baking soda with 10 drops of lemon or orange, 5 drops of tea tree, 5 drops of lemongrass, and 10 drops of lavender oil. Mix these and sprinkle the mixture over your carpets. Next, use a dry brush or a sponge on your carpets to rub the mixture so it goes in deep into the carpet bottom.

Allow this mixture to sit for 2 hours and then vacuum out the mixture. The process may be lengthy, but the results are long-lasting and worth the effort. Do this at least once a month.

- **Removing Scrum from Shower Curtain**

When water interacts with dirt, soap, and other substances during your shower, a dark and filmy bacterial line begins to form. Not only it's disgusting but mold and mildew build-up over time also cause infections and diseases. Do away with harsh, commercial products and reach out for a spray bottle with warm water and add in 4 drops of clove, tea tree oil, and eucalyptus oil. Spray these into your shower surface and let it sit for a few minutes. Take your scrub brush and watch the mold, mildew, and scrum easily come off, leaving your floors and walls clean.

Personal Care

- **Keep Flying Bugs Away**

Summer is great, but what isn't so great are the bugs that come out in full force. These outdoor pests are a nuisance, but what's even worse is using dangerous chemical-laden bug sprays and repellents. Why not make your own version of bug repellents that are less harmful and more affordable?

Here is a great recipe you can try. In a small spray bottle, fill it up with distilled water and add 1.5 ounces of vodka or witch hazel. Put 30 drops of lemongrass essential oil into this mixture. Mix your bottle so everything inside is well-combined. You can spray this mixture onto outdoor furniture, walls, and floors to ward off mosquitoes, flies, and other pesky insects for you to have a bug-free, chemical-free barbeque.

- **Soothe Pain**

Most people pop an aspirin or some kind of over-the-counter medication to suppress their headache. However, if you have a few bottles of essential oils, why not create your own all-natural pain medication?

All you need is almond oil combined with 4 drops of peppermint essential oils, 2 drops of rosemary, 4 drops of peppermint, and 1 drop of lavender essential oil. If you like, you can also add in some frankincense and chamomile essential oil. Put this in a bottle and shake it up. Each time you have a headache or even feel stressed out, apply this mixture on your pulse points, temples, and the back of your neck. Close your eyes and breathe in the scent.

- **Make Your Own Hand Sanitizer**

Antibacterial hand sanitizers can be quite dangerous, and if you are put off by the alcoholic smell of certain sanitizers, you can create your very own one that smells amazing and is safe. Start by infusing organic aloe vera gel with 10 drops of tea tree oil and 5-7 drops of lavender essential oil. Pour this into a glass bottle–not plastic—because glass bottles allow the mixture to stay fresh longer. Use this as your on-the-go sanitizer.

- **Ease Your Aching Muscles**

Massage therapists usually incorporate essential oils into their massages because it has many soothing properties and effects on the body. Essential oils not only soothe your muscles but also helps with sleep, relaxation, and pain relief. If you find yourself having aches in certain parts of your body due to exercise, sitting too much, or having unnecessary cramps, combine a ½ ounce of grapeseed oil in a small glass bottle as your carrier oil and add in about 8-10 drops of peppermint, lavender, and eucalyptus oil. Shake the bottle and rub this on the places that you feel the ache so you have added relaxation and comfort.

- **Soften and Grow Your Hair**

Everybody loves soft and shiny hair. Melaleuca oil has been used for thousands of years to maintain and promote natural, healthy hair. It has strong antiseptic and antifungal elements which make this oil extremely effective at treating dandruff, head lice, and itchy scalp.

Essential oil has also helped hair growth among patients with alopecia. For smooth and shiny hair, you can try adding several drops of melaleuca oil into your hair conditioner and use it as you normally do by massaging it into your scalp.

- **Clean Makeup Brushes**

Washing your makeup brushes is an essential and extremely important step in your makeup routine. Regular use of your brushes without any cleaning can lead to bacterial growth and buildup. Store-bought cleaners are no doubt pricey and, of course, chemical-laden.

By combining 2 tablespoons of witch hazel with ½ teaspoon of extra virgin olive oil, 20 drops of tea tree essential oil, and 2 teaspoons of castile soap, you now have your very own antifungal makeup brush cleaner. You can double this recipe and keep it in a glass bottle. Whenever you clean your brushes, pour in a certain amount into a bowl and swirl your brushes inside the mixture until the makeup residue and dirt are removed. Once you're done, rinse your brushes with water, clean out your bowl, and squeeze out any excess liquid in the brushes. Set them out to dry.

Chapter 9: Using Essential Oils for General Health

Essential oils are more than just nice-smelling oils. By now, you already know the different benefits of essentials oils. In this chapter, we will look at its benefits on increasing our energy, on improving our digestion, as well as helping increase our emotional health.

Here are some ways you can use different essential oils for various needs. Keep in mind that if you want to make these oils, you should store them in amber bottles to prevent oxidation and also to keep them fresh longer. These bottles can be stored in a cool place, away from sunlight.

Essentials Oils for Better Health

- *Joint and Cartilage Pain Relief*

Add 2 tablespoons of fractionated coconut oil with 12 drops patchouli oil, 10 drops marjoram oil, 9 drops lemongrass oil, and 9 drops juniper berry oil. Apply when needed to relieve the pain.

- *Anti-Inflammatory Lotion*

Mix 7 drops each of patchouli and ylang-ylang oil, 6 drops each of chamomile and ginger oil, and 2 drops of myrrh oil. Pour mixture into your favorite lotion and mix until well-blended. Pour contents into a lotion bottle to use.

- *Fibromyalgia Pain*

Mix fractionated coconut oil with 20 drops each of chamomile, lavender, marjoram, and orange essential oil. Fill a rollerball bottle with the mixture and apply whenever needed.

- *Sciatica Support*

Fill a rollerball bottle with 7 drops each of nutmeg, marjoram, and chamomile oil, and 4 drops lavender oil. Apply as often as needed.

- *Ligament Tear Blend*

Mix 5 drops lemongrass and 15 drops lavender together. Use hot compress to apply to skin. Do this at least 3 times a day to aid muscle and ligament recovery.

- *Tendonitis Blend*

Mix 4 drops each of allspice berry, basil, and bay oil, and apply to affected area with a hot compress.

Essential Oils for Emotional Well-being

For some people, an emotional boost can be things like retail therapy or even a hair wash or eating a big tub of ice cream. All of these things are great, but we can't be doing this all the time. For a more holistic approach to emotional health and well-being, here are some essential oil recipes that you can do while at home to boost your emotions and keep you calm and peaceful. These blends can even be added to your diffuser and can be kept at your workstation for times when you feel a quick pick-me-up.

- *The Mood-Boosting Spritz*

In a spritz bottle, mix 2 drops of bergamot oil with 3 drops each of lemon and orange essential oils. Top the bottle with sparkling water and spritz anytime you feel you need a mood booster.

- *The Stress Relief Balm*

In a glass balm container, whip 2 tablespoons of fractionated coconut oil. Add in rosemary, lavender, and sage essential oils. Mix well and pour contents into balm container and use whenever necessary.

- **_Romance Diffuser_**

Add a romantic touch to your candlelight dinner by adding 3 drops each of jasmine, sandalwood, and rose essential oils into the diffuser.

- **_Focusing Concoction_**

For times when you need to concentrate, add in 3 drops each of rosemary and cinnamon essential oils in a diffuser and set in your office, study room, or workroom.

- **_For a Calming Balance_**

This is a great way of adding some essential oils to your office space. Mix dried potpourri with orange, patchouli, and ginger essential oils and let steep for one week in a dark and dry area. Once done, place potpourri in small bags and keep in places like your car and vanity desk.

- *Christmas Time of the Year*

To ring in the holiday season, add in essential oils of fir, cedarwood, and orange into your diffuser.

- *Blissful Soak*

Fill your bathtub with hot water. Add in a few drops of orange, grapefruit, rosemary, lemon, and bergamot essential oils together with 5 cups of Epsom salt. When the water is slightly warm to touch, sink in for a relaxing soak.

- *Beating Depression*

Set your diffuser and add in 5 drops each of geranium, sage, lemon, and jasmine essential oils. Do this as often as you like.

- *Anxiety Fighter*

To beat anxiety, keep a rollerball container filled with sandalwood, cedarwood,
Bergamot, frankincense, and ylang-ylang essential oils. Rub this at different pressure points like your temples, your wrists, and behind your earlobe for an instant relaxer.

- **For Post-Traumatic Stress Disorder (PTSD)**

Make a balm by mixing fractionated coconut oil together with lemongrass, sandalwood, cedarwood, jasmine, sage, and chamomile essential oils. Rub on temples and ears to combat PTSD.

- **Aiding Autism**

Lavender, patchouli, and anise essential oils mixed together can help reduce symptoms of autism. You can use this combination in a diffuser or even in a rollerball bottle. Apply whenever necessary.

- **Addiction Help**

If you or someone you know is suffering from any kind of addiction, black pepper, clove, anise, cinnamon, and grapefruit are all good essential oils to help curb this problem. Mix these and pour it into an inhaler.

- **Motivating Blend**

To lift your spirits and motivate you, mix 2 drops each of black pepper, lime, orange, and frankincense essential oils into a rollerball container and apply whenever required.

- *Anxiety Aid*

If you suffer from frequent bouts of anxiety, add a calming blend of anise, bergamot, cinnamon, and lavender essential oils into an inhaler. Inhale to slow down your breathing and pulse to make you more relaxed.

- *Recovering from a Loss*

You can either do this in a diffuser or a bath soak. Mix geranium, sandalwood, lavender, marjoram, and some orange essential oil. These oils can help soothe emotional responses during a time of grief.

Essential Oils for Overall Quality of Life

Using essential oils for common ailments or just having a few bottles of your favorite mixture around for coughs, cold, bacterial infection, and so on is one of the ways we can enhance our daily life for the better. This is because we reduce the need to buy store-bought enhancers or perfumes or medication to make ourselves feel better. Essential oils are also cheaper.

- *Fearfulness*

To reduce fear and increase confidence, create a blend of cedarwood, anise, sandalwood, and jasmine essential oils.

Pour this blend into a rollerball container and apply on the nape of the neck, behind the ears, and on the wrists.

- **Acid Reflux**

Fill up a vegetable capsule with peppermint oil. Take two whenever you feel discomfort. You can also massage your stomach with peppermint oil if your symptoms are mild.

- **Asthma**

Diffusing lavender and orange essential oils daily in your home will help alleviate symptoms experienced by people living with asthma. Alternatively, these essential oils can also be included into an inhaler for mobile use.

- **Bacterial Infection**

For simple infections like a cut on the arm or even on the toenail, mix peppermint, sage, and cinnamon essential oils. Either apply this directly to the affected area as often as possible or apply it to the liver area of the body. You can even apply it to the soles of your feet.

- ***Bee Sting***

Provided that you did not get stung badly or in areas that prohibit breathing, a quick application of basil and chamomile essential oils together with a cold compress will help alleviate the symptoms of a bee sting.

- **Bronchitis**

Eucalyptus, thyme, and basil essential oils, either diffused or inhaled, will also help alleviate symptoms of bronchitis and help the sufferer breathe better over time.

- ***Burns***

If you have a minor burn, a mixture of lavender and geranium essential oils applied to the affected area will help cool the skin and aid in the healing process. Apply this mixture regularly until the scar has healed.

Chapter 10: Easy-to-follow Recipes for Several Health-Related Concerns

Stress

Relieve that stress.

Supplies that you will need:

Lavender Essential Oil

Lemon Bark Essential Oil

Clary Sage Essential Oil

Glass dram that is equipped with a spout for blending

Purified Water

Directions for blending:

1. In order to prepare this blend properly, you will need to have a glass dram to use for preparation prior to placing it in the diffuser. Start with the Clary Sage oil by applying 3 drops into the dram.
2. Then, add in the Lavender and Lemon Oil by applying 1 drop each into the dram, and then blend properly.
3. Pour the purified water into the diffuser, and then add your oil blend.

4. Turn on the diffuser and enjoy.

No more stress.

Supplies that you will need:

Vetiver Essential Oil

Lavender Essential Oil

Roman Chamomile Essential Oil

Glass dram that is equipped with a spout for blending

Purified Water

Directions for blending:

1. In order to prepare this blend properly, you will need to have a glass dram to use for preparation prior to placing it in the diffuser. Start with the Lavender and Roman Chamomile oil applying 2 drops into the dram.
2. Then, add in the Vetiver Oil applying 1 drop into the dram and blend properly.
3. Pour the purified water into the diffuser and then add your oil blend.
4. Turn on the diffuser and enjoy.

Reduction of Stress

Supplies that you will need:

Allspice Essential Oil

Purified Water

Melissa Essential Oils

Glass dram that is equipped with a spout for blending

Directions for blending:

1. In order to prepare this blend properly, you will need to have a glass dram to use for preparation prior to placing it in the roller bottle. Start with the Allspice and Melissa Oil and drop 10 drops into the dram.
2. Roll the dram in the palms of your hands to blend the oils together.
3. Pour in the purified water and then add your oil blend into the diffuser with the water.
4. Turn on the diffuser and enjoy.

To apply:

Pour the purified water into the diffuser and add in the essential oil blend. Then, turn on the diffuser and enjoy the essential oils throughout your home. This will create a stress reduced environment.

Stress be gone.

Supplies that you will need:

Frankincense Essential Oil

Sweet Orange Essential Oil

Lavender Essential Oil

Glass dram that is equipped with a spout for blending
Purified Water

Directions for blending:

1. In order to prepare this blend properly, you will need to have a glass dram to use for preparation prior to placing it in the diffuser. Start with the Lavender and Frankincense oil applying 3 drops into the dram.
2. Then, add in the Sweet Orange applying 1 drop into the dram and blend properly.
3. Pour the purified water into the diffuser and then add your oil blend.
4. Turn on the diffuser and enjoy.

Anxiety

Supplies that you will need:

Bergamot Essential Oil
Lavender Essential Oil
Clary Sage Essential Oil
Glass dram that is equipped with a spout for blending
Purified Water

Directions for blending:

1. In order to prepare this blend properly, you will need to have a glass dram to use for preparation prior to

placing it in the diffuser. Start with the Lavender and Clary Sage oil applying 2 drops into the dram.

2. Then, add in the Bergamot Oil applying 1 drop into the dram and blend properly.

3. Pour the purified water into the diffuser and then add your oil blend.

4. Turn on the diffuser and enjoy.

Anxiety Blend

Supplies that you will need:

Patchouli Essential Oil

Ylang-Ylang Essential Oil

Geranium Essential Oil

Clary Sage Essential Oil

Glass dram that is equipped with a spout for blending

Purified Water

Directions for blending:

1. In order to prepare this blend properly, you will need to have a glass dram to use for preparation prior to placing it in the diffuser. Start with the Clary Sage and Geranium oil applying 2 drops into the dram.

2. Then, add in the Ylang-Ylang and Patchouli applying 1 drop each the dram and blend properly.

3. Pour the purified water into the diffuser and then add your oil blend.

4. Turn on the diffuser and enjoy.

Anxious Blend

Supplies that you will need:
Patchouli Essential Oil
Wild Orange Essential Oil
Cedarwood Essential Oil
Ylang-Ylang Essential Oil
Glass dram that is equipped with a spout for blending
Purified Water

Directions for blending:

1. In order to prepare this blend properly, you will need to have a glass dram to use for preparation prior to placing it in the diffuser. Start with the Wild Orange and Cedarwood oil applying 2 drops into the dram.
2. Then, add in the Patchouli and Ylang-Ylang applying 1 drop each into the dram and blend properly.
3. Pour the purified water into the diffuser and then add your oil blend.
4. Turn on the diffuser and enjoy.

Depression

Happily, wake up.

Supplies that you will need:
Ylang-Ylang Essential Oil

Bergamot Essential Oil

Glass dram that is equipped with a spout for blending

Purified Water

Directions for blending:

1. In order to prepare this blend properly, you will need to have a glass dram to use for preparation prior to placing it in the diffuser. Start with the Bergamot and the Ylang-Ylang oil applying 3 drops into the dram.
2. Pour the purified water into the diffuser and then add your oil blend.
3. Turn on the diffuser and enjoy.

Elevate your moods.

Supplies that you will need:

Geranium Essential Oil

Orange Essential Oil

Allspice Essential Oil

Bergamot Essential Oil

Glass dram that is equipped with a spout for blending

Purified Water

Diffuser

Directions for blending:

1. In order to prepare this blend properly, you will need to have a glass dram to use for preparation prior to

placing it in the glass spray bottle. Start with the Geranium Oil and drop 5 drops into the dram.

2. Then, use the Bergamot Oil and drop in 4 drops.

3. Next, pour some Orange Oil, and Allspice Oil into the dram. You will need 3 drops.

4. Roll the dram in the palms of your hands to blend the oils together.

5. Once you have poured in your blended essential oils, place the 4 fluid ounces of water into the diffuser and pour in the oil blend.

6. Turn on your diffuser and let the oil do its magic.

To apply:

This blend will increase your mood and also help you to elevate the moods of others in the same vicinity. Bergamot is known as a natural anti-depressant. This can increase the moods of children as well as those that suffer from depression.

Uplift your moods.

Supplies that you will need:

Clove Essential Oil

Patchouli Essential Oils

Rose Essential Oil

Geranium Essential Oil

Glass dram that is equipped with a spout for blending

Glass container with a sealable lid

Your favorite carrier oils

Directions for blending:

1. In order to prepare this blend properly, you will need to have a glass dram to use for preparation prior to placing it in the glass storage container. Start with the Rose oil by dropping 5 drops into the dram.
2. Then, place the Patchouli, and Geranium into the container with 4 drops each.
3. Next, place your Clove Oil into the dram with 2 drops.
4. Roll the dram in the palms of your hands to blend the oils together.
5. Then, pour into your storage container that is glass.
6. Once you have poured in your blended essential oils, use your carrier oil and pour in 1 tsp of oil.
7. Place the lid on the storage container and roll the container between your hands a couple of times, then rotate the bottle using your first finger and thumb in an up-down motion.
8. This will help the oils to blend properly.

To apply:

Ensure that you are not allergic to any of the ingredients found in this recipe. When you are feeling a need for your spirits to be lifted, apply this oil blend to your back, the back of your neck, and your chest for an uplifting experience. This will help with combatting those blues.

Mountain Top Wake Up

Supplies that you will need:
Ylang-Ylang Essential Oil
Idaho Balsam Fir Essential Oil
Glass dram that is equipped with a spout for blending
Purified Water

Directions for blending:

1. In order to prepare this blend properly, you will need to have a glass dram to use for preparation prior to placing it in the diffuser. Start with the Ylang-Ylang and the Idaho Balsam Fir applying 3 drops into the dram.
2. Pour the purified water into the diffuser and then add your oil blend.
3. Turn on the diffuser and enjoy.

Energy Boosting

Boosting Your Energy #1

Supplies that you will need:
Lemon Essential Oil
Peppermint Essential Oil

Frankincense Essential Oil

Glass dram that is equipped with a spout for blending

Purified Water

Directions for blending:

1. In order to prepare this blend properly, you will need to have a glass dram to use for preparation prior to placing it in the diffuser. Start with the Frankincense, Lemon, and Peppermint oil applying 2 drops into the dram and blending properly.
2. Pour the purified water into the diffuser and then add your oil blend.
3. Turn on the diffuser and enjoy.

Boosting Your Energy #2

Supplies that you will need:

Rosemary Essential Oil

Black Pepper Essential Oil

Glass dram that is equipped with a spout for blending

Purified Water

Directions for blending:

1. In order to prepare this blend properly, you will need to have a glass dram to use for preparation prior to placing it in the diffuser. Start with the Rosemary and

Black Pepper oil applying 3 drops into the dram and blending properly.

2. Pour the purified water into the diffuser and then add your oil blend.
3. Turn on the diffuser and enjoy.

Boosting Your Energy #3

Supplies that you will need:

Lemon Essential Oil

Cinnamon Bark Essential Oil

Grapefruit Essential Oil

Sweet Orange Essential Oil

Glass dram that is equipped with a spout for blending

Purified Water

Directions for blending:

1. In order to prepare this blend properly, you will need to have a glass dram to use for preparation prior to placing it in the diffuser. Start with the Lemon, Sweet Orange and Grapefruit oil applying 5 drops into the dram.
2. Then, add in the Cinnamon Bark applying 2 drops into the dram and blend properly.
3. Pour the purified water into the diffuser and then add your oil blend.
4. Turn on the diffuser and enjoy.

Chapter 11: Easy-to-Follow Recipes for Women's Issues

Menopause

Supplies that you will need:

Rosemary Essential Oil

Ylang-Ylang Essential Oil

Geranium Essential Oil

Lavender Essential Oil

Rose Otto Essential Oil

Roman Chamomile Essential Oil

Peppermint Essential Oil

Glass dram that is equipped with a spout for blending

Purified Water

Directions for blending:

1. In order to prepare this blend properly, you will need to have a glass dram to use for preparation prior to placing it in the diffuser. Start with the Geranium, Lavender, and Rosemary oil applying 20 drops into the dram.

2. Then, add in the Peppermint, Ylang-Ylang, Rose Otto and Chamomile Oil applying 10 drops into the dram and blend properly.

3. Pour the purified water into the diffuser and then add 10 drops of your oil blend for each diffuser use.
4. Turn on the diffuser and enjoy.

Menopause No More

Supplies that you will need:

Lavender Essential Oil

Peppermint Essential Oil

Aloe Vera Gel

Glass dram that is equipped with a spout for blending

Purified Water

Glass spray bottle

Directions for blending:

1. In order to prepare this blend properly, you will need to have a glass dram to use for preparation prior to placing it in the diffuser. Start with the Peppermint and lavender oil applying 5 drops into the dram.
2. Then, add in the 1 tsp Aloe Vera gel and 1 cup of distilled water.
3. Pour the purified water into the glass spray bottle and then add your oil blend.
4. Spritz your face when dealing with hot flashes to cool down the body.

Meno-Paus

Supplies that you will need:

Ylang-Ylang Essential Oil

Bergamot Essential Oil

Geranium Essential Oil

Sandalwood Essential Oil

Clary Sage Essential Oil

Rose Otto Essential Oil

Coconut Oil-Fractionated

Glass dram that is equipped with a spout for blending

Rollerball container that is 10 mL-glass

Directions for blending:

1. In order to prepare this blend properly, you will need to have a glass dram to use for preparation prior to placing it in the diffuser. Start with the Rose Otto and Clary Sage oil applying 10 drops into the dram.

2. Then, add in the Geranium, Ylang-Ylang, Sandalwood, and Bergamot applying 5 drops each into the dram and blend properly.

3. Pour the oils into the roller ball container and then add in the coconut oil.

4. Apply to your ankles, feet, the bottom of your stomach and wrists once a day.

Menstrual cramps

Cramps from PMS

Supplies that you will need:

Geranium Essential Oil

Lavender Essential Oil

Clary Sage Essential Oil

Avocado oil

Glass dram that is equipped with a spout for blending

Rollerball container 10 mL- glass

Directions for blending:

1. In order to prepare this blend properly, you will need to have a glass dram to use for preparation prior to placing it in the diffuser. Start with the Clary Sage oil applying 3 drops into the dram.

2. Then, add in the Lavender applying 2 drops into the dram and blend properly.

3. Next, add in the Geranium using 1 drop. Blend it together and place in the roller ball container.

4. Then, fill the container with the avocado oil.

5. Massage the oil on the abdomen once daily for PMS symptoms.

PMS Relief

Supplies that you will need:

Cypress Essential Oil

Lavender Essential Oil

Peppermint Essential Oil

Jojoba

Glass dram that is equipped with a spout for blending

Glass roller container

Directions for blending:

1. In order to prepare this blend properly, you will need to have a glass dram to use for preparation prior to placing it in the diffuser. Start with the Peppermint oil applying 5 drops into the dram.

2. Then, add in the Cypress Oil applying 4 drops into the dram and blend properly.

3. Next, add the lavender oil applying 3 drops into the dram.

4. Once blended pour into roller container and add the Jojoba oil.

5. Massage into those small abdominal areas that are cramping once per day.

Pre-Menstrual Symptoms Relief

Supplies that you will need:

Lavender Essential Oil

Lemon Essential Oil

Peppermint Essential Oil

Epsom Salt

Whole Milk

Glass dram that is equipped with a spout for blending

Directions for blending:

1. In order to prepare this blend properly, you will need to have a glass dram to use for preparation prior to placing it in the diffuser. Start with the Lemon, Lavender and Peppermint oil applying 10 drops into the dram.
2. Run your bath, then pour Epsom salt (2cups) allowing it to dissolve.
3. Next, pour your mixed essential oils into the 2 cups of whole milk. Then, pour it into the bath.
4. Relax in the bath for 15 minutes for a fully immersive therapeutic bath.

Headaches

Boo on Headaches

Supplies that you will need:

Lavender Essential Oil

Eucalyptus Essential Oil

Rosemary Essential Oil

Peppermint Essential oil

Glass dram that is equipped with a spout for blending
Purified Water

Directions for blending:

1. In order to prepare this blend properly, you will need to have a glass dram to use for preparation prior to placing it in the diffuser. Start with the Lavender and Peppermint oil applying 2 drops into the dram.
2. Then, add in the Rosemary and Eucalyptus applying 1 drop each into the dram and blend properly.
3. Pour the purified water into the diffuser and then add your oil blend.
4. Turn on the diffuser and enjoy.

Stress Headache

Supplies that you will need:

Peppermint Essential Oil
Lavender Essential Oil
Thyme Essential Oil
Sweet Marjoram Essential oil
Rosemary Essential Oil
Glass dram that is equipped with a spout for blending
Purified Water

Directions for blending:

1. In order to prepare this blend properly, you will need to have a glass dram to use for preparation prior to placing it in the diffuser. Start with the Lavender, Sweet Marjoram, thyme, Peppermint and Rosemary oil applying 2 drops into the dram.
2. Pour the purified water into the diffuser and then add your oil blend.
3. Turn on the diffuser and enjoy.

Headache Sinus Cavity

Supplies that you will need:

Basil Essential Oil

Peppermint Essential Oil

Frankincense Essential Oil

Lavender Essential oil

Glass dram that is equipped with a spout for blending

Purified Water

Directions for blending:

1. In order to prepare this blend properly, you will need to have a glass dram to use for preparation prior to placing it in the diffuser. Start with the Lavender and Peppermint oil applying 4 drops into the dram.
2. Then, add in the Basil and Frankincense applying 2 drops into the dram and blend properly.

3. Pour the purified water into the diffuser and then add your oil blend.
4. Turn on the diffuser and enjoy.

Morning Sickness

Bust that nausea.

Supplies that you will need:

Grapefruit Essential Oil

Lime Essential Oil

Spearmint Essential Oil

Sweet Orange Essential oil

Glass dram that is equipped with a spout for blending

Purified Water

Directions for blending:

1. In order to prepare this blend properly, you will need to have a glass dram to use for preparation prior to placing it in the diffuser. Start with the Grapefruit, Sweet Orange, Spearmint, and Lime oil applying 1 drop into the dram.
2. Pour the purified water into the diffuser and then add your oil blend.
3. Turn on the diffuser and enjoy.

Anti-Nausea Oil Blend

Supplies that you will need:

Lavender Essential Oil

Peppermint Essential Oil

Carrier Oil of your choice

Glass dram that is equipped with a spout for blending

Directions for blending:

1. In order to prepare this blend properly, you will need to have a glass dram to use for preparation prior to placing it in the diffuser. Start with the lavender oil applying 10 drops and Peppermint Oil applying 5 drops into the dram.

2. Then, blend it with the 30 mL of your favorite carrier oil. Use one that does not make you sick to your stomach.

3. Sniff this from an inhaler or place a few drops on your hands and breath it in when feeling sick.

No More Sickness

Supplies that you will need:

Lemon Essential Oil

Peppermint Essential Oil

Glass dram that is equipped with a spout for blending

Carrier Oil

Directions for blending:

1. In order to prepare this blend properly, you will need to have a glass dram to use for preparation prior to placing it in the diffuser. Start with the Lemon oil applying 8 drops into the dram.
2. Then, add in the Peppermint Oil applying 7 drops into the dram and blend properly.
3. Then, pour it into a glass bottle with about 30 mL of your favorite carrier oil that does not make you sick.
4. Sniff this bottle or drip a bit into your hands and sniff your hands when feeling sick.

Ginger-block this nausea.

Supplies that you will need:

Ginger Essential Oil

Chamomile Essential Oil

Peppermint Essential Oil

Glass dram that is equipped with a spout for blending

Carrier Oil

Directions for blending:

1. In order to prepare this blend properly, you will need to have a glass dram to use for preparation prior to placing it in the diffuser. Start with the Peppermint, ginger, and Chamomile oil applying 10 drops into the dram.

2. Next, mix it in a bottle with the carrier oil that does not make your sick.

3. Use this to sniff or apply to a handkerchief and sniff them when feeling sick. Do not use direct topical application. It can cause burning.

Chapter 12: Easy-to-Follow Recipes for Everyday Living

Enhance Your Skin and Beauty Routine.

Grow me some hair.

Supplies that you will need:

Lavender Essential Oil

Peppermint Bark Essential Oil

Cedarwood Essential Oil

Rosemary Essential Oil

Glass dram that is equipped with a spout for blending

Coconut Oil

Castor Oil Jamaican Black

Directions for blending:

1. In order to prepare this blend properly, you will need to have a glass dram to use for preparation prior to placing it in the diffuser. Start with the Peppermint, rosemary, Lavender, and Cedarwood oil applying 10 drops into the dram.

2. Then, add in the coconut oil and the castor oil that is Jamaican Black in ¼ cup increments.

3. Blend properly and then apply to your hair to stimulate the follicles to grow.

Perfect Facial

Supplies that you will need:

Frankincense Essential Oil

Hazelnut carrier Oil

Rose Essential Oil

Jasmine Essential Oil

Glass dram that is equipped with a spout for blending

Directions for blending:

1. In order to prepare this blend properly, you will need to have a glass dram to use for preparation prior to placing it in the diffuser. Start with the Jasmine, Rose and Frankincense oil applying 10 drops into the dram.
2. Next, add in the Hazelnut carrier oil using 2 tbsps. of oil.
3. Blend it together completely and apply to your face after you have pre-washed your face.

Oily Skin Facial

Supplies that you will need:

Lemon Essential Oil

Petitgrain Essential Oil

Orange Essential Oil

Grapeseed Carrier Oil

Glass dram that is equipped with a spout for blending

Directions for blending:

1. In order to prepare this blend properly, you will need to have a glass dram to use for preparation prior to placing it in the diffuser. Start with the Petitgrain, Lemon, and Orange oil applying 10 drops into the dram.

2. Next, add in the Grapeseed carrier oil using 2 tbsps. of oil.

3. Blend it together completely and apply to your face after you have pre-washed your face.

Problem Skin Facial

Supplies that you will need:

Bois De Rose Essential Oil

Lavender Essential Oil

Myrrh Essential Oil

chamomile Essential Oil

KuKui nut Carrier Oil

Glass dram that is equipped with a spout for blending

Directions for blending:

1. In order to prepare this blend properly, you will need to have a glass dram to use for preparation prior to placing it in the diffuser. Start with the Chamomile and Myrrh oil applying 10 drops into the dram.

2. Then, add in the Lavender and Bois De Rose applying 5 drops into the dram and blend properly.

3. Next, add in the KuKui Nut carrier oil using 2 tbsps. of oil.

4. Blend it together completely and apply to your face after you have pre-washed your face.

Cure Ailments in Your Family.

Bug Repellent

Supplies that you will need:

Citronella Essential Oil

Lemongrass Essential Oil

Glass dram that is equipped with a spout for blending

Directions for blending:

1. In order to prepare this blend properly, you will need to have a glass dram to use for preparation prior to placing it in the diffuser. Start with the Citronella and lemongrass oil applying 3 drops into the dram.
2. Once blended properly, pour it into a spray bottle and prior to heading outside spray everyone. This will keep the bugs away while outside.

Clear those bronchi's.

Supplies that you will need:

Myrrh Essential Oil

Frankincense Essential Oil

Ravensara Essential Oil

Sage Essential Oil

Clove Essential Oil

Glass dram that is equipped with a spout for blending

Carrier oil of your choice

Directions for blending:

1. In order to prepare this blend properly, you will need to have a glass dram to use for preparation prior to placing it in the diffuser. Start with the Frankincense oil applying 15 drops into the dram.

2. Then, add in the Ravensara applying 6 drops into the dram and blend properly.

3. Next, add Clove Oil using 5 drops, as well as Myrrh oil with 4 drops and Sage Oil with 2 drops into the dram.

4. Blend until fully blended. Then, pour into a glass container for storage.

5. Mix in the carrier oil of your choice using 1 tbsp.

6. Apply to the back, the chest, and the neck up to 3 times a day.

Influenza No-No

Supplies that you will need:

Oregano Essential Oil

Ravensara Essential Oil

Thyme Essential Oil

Clove Essential oil

Hyssop Essential Oil

Cinnamon Leaf Essential Oil

Glass dram that is equipped with a spout for blending

Purified water

Directions for blending:

1. In order to prepare this blend properly, you will need to have a glass dram to use for preparation prior to placing it in the diffuser. Start with the Ravensara oil applying 10 drops into the dram.

2. Then, add in the Oregano applying 8 drops into the dram and blend properly.

3. Next, apply the cinnamon leaf using 7 drops, the thyme using 6 drops, the hyssop using 5 drops and the clove using 4 drops.

4. Pour this into a storage container and then use 5-20 drips per diffuser session.

5. Pour the purified water into the diffuser and then add your oil blend.

6. Turn on the diffuser and enjoy.

Pneumonia Go Away

Supplies that you will need:

Oregano Essential Oil

Peppermint Essential Oil

Frankincense Essential Oil

Rosemary Essential Oil

Ravensara Essential Oil

Glass dram that is equipped with a spout for blending

Rollerball container

Carrier Oil

Directions for blending:

1. In order to prepare this blend properly, you will need to have a glass dram to use for preparation prior to placing it in the diffuser. Start with the Rosemary oil applying 10 drops into the dram.
2. Then, add in the Frankincense and Ravensara applying 8 drops into the dram and blend properly.
3. Next, apply the Peppermint and Hyssop oil using 2 drops to the dram.
4. Now, add it all to the carrier oil using 1 tbsp. and apply it 3 times per day on the chest and neck.

Spruce Up Your Home.

Home is balanced.

Supplies that you will need:

Juniper Berry Essential Oil

Lavender Essential Oil

Bergamot Essential Oil

Glass dram that is equipped with a spout for blending

Purified Water

Directions for blending:

1. In order to prepare this blend properly, you will need to have a glass dram to use for preparation prior to placing it in the diffuser. Start with the Bergamot and lavender oil applying 2 drops into the dram.

2. Then, add in the Juniper Berry applying 1 drop into the dram and blend properly.

3. Pour the purified water into the diffuser and then add your oil blend.

4. Turn on the diffuser and enjoy.

Sea Breeze

Supplies that you will need:

Tangerine Essential Oil

Cypress Essential Oil

Arborvitae Essential Oil

Glass dram that is equipped with a spout for blending

Purified Water

Directions for blending:

1. In order to prepare this blend properly, you will need to have a glass dram to use for preparation prior to placing it in the diffuser. Start with the Tangerine and Cypress oil applying 3 drops into the dram.
2. Then, add in the Arborville applying 2 drops into the dram and blend properly.
3. Pour the purified water into the diffuser and then add your oil blend.
4. Turn on the diffuser and enjoy.

Air is clean.

Supplies that you will need:

Tangerine Essential Oil

Eucalyptus Essential Oil

Lavender Essential Oil

Glass dram that is equipped with a spout for blending

Purified Water

Directions for blending:

1. In order to prepare this blend properly, you will need to have a glass dram to use for preparation prior to placing it in the diffuser. Start with the Tangerine and lavender oil applying 3 drops into the dram.

2. Then, add in the Eucalyptus applying 2 drops into the dram and blend properly.

3. Pour the purified water into the diffuser and then add your oil blend.

4. Turn on the diffuser and enjoy.

Home is the heart of everyone.

Supplies that you will need:

Orange Essential Oil

Cinnamon Essential Oil

Lemon Essential Oil

Glass dram that is equipped with a spout for blending

Purified Water

Directions for blending:

1. In order to prepare this blend properly, you will need to have a glass dram to use for preparation prior to placing it in the diffuser. Start with the Cinnamon, Orange, and Lemon oil applying 3 drops into the dram.
2. Pour the purified water into the diffuser and then add your oil blend.
3. Turn on the diffuser and enjoy.

Delight in Your Home

Supplies that you will need:

Tea Tree Essential Oil

Spearmint Essential Oil

Lime Essential Oil

Glass dram that is equipped with a spout for blending

Purified Water

Directions for blending:

1. In order to prepare this blend properly, you will need to have a glass dram to use for preparation prior to placing it in the diffuser. Start with the Lime oil applying 3 drops into the dram.
2. Then, add in the Spearmint and Tea Tree oil using 2 drops each.
3. Pour the purified water into the diffuser and then add your oil blend.
4. Turn on the diffuser and enjoy.

Pumpkin Spice

Supplies that you will need:

Orange Essential Oil

Thieves Essential Oil

Glass dram that is equipped with a spout for blending

Purified Water

Directions for blending:

1. In order to prepare this blend properly, you will need to have a glass dram to use for preparation prior to placing it in the diffuser. Start with the Orange and thieves oil applying 3 drops into the dram.
2. Pour the purified water into the diffuser and then add your oil blend.
3. Turn on the diffuser and enjoy.

Holiday Delight Apples

Supplies that you will need:

Ginger Essential Oil

Cinnamon Essential Oil

Orange Essential Oil

Glass dram that is equipped with a spout for blending

Purified Water

Directions for blending:

1. In order to prepare this blend properly, you will need to have a glass dram to use for preparation prior to placing it in the diffuser. Start with the Orange oil applying 4 drops into the dram.
2. Then, add in the Ginger and Cinnamon Oil using 2 drops of oil in the dram.
3. Pour the purified water into the diffuser and then add your oil blend.
4. Turn on the diffuser and enjoy.

Christmas Fur

Supplies that you will need:

Idaho Balsam Fir Essential Oil

Pine Essential Oil

Idaho Blue Spruce Essential Oil

Glass dram that is equipped with a spout for blending

Purified Water

Directions for blending:

1. In order to prepare this blend properly, you will need to have a glass dram to use for preparation prior to placing it in the diffuser. Start with the Pine, Idaho Balsam Fir, and the Idaho Blue Spruce oil applying 2 drops into the dram.
2. Pour the purified water into the diffuser and then add your oil blend.
3. Turn on the diffuser and enjoy.

Put the kids to bed.

Supplies that you will need:

Orange Essential Oil

Cedarwood Essential Oil

Glass dram that is equipped with a spout for blending

Purified Water

Directions for blending:

1. In order to prepare this blend properly, you will need to have a glass dram to use for preparation prior to placing it in the diffuser. Start with the Cedarwood and orange oil applying 3 drops into the dram.
2. Pour the purified water into the diffuser and then add your oil blend.
3. Turn on the diffuser and enjoy.

Fighting Demons in Your Sleep

Supplies that you will need:

Hawaiian Sandalwood Essential Oil

Ylang-Ylang Essential Oil

Bergamot Essential Oil

Juniper Essential Oil

Vetiver Essential Oil

Rose Essential Oil

Lavender Essential Oil

Tangerine Essential Oil

Glass dram that is equipped with a spout for blending

Purified Water

Directions for blending:

1. In order to prepare this blend properly, you will need to have a glass dram to use for preparation prior to placing it in the diffuser. Start with the addition of all the available oils listed above.
2. Pour the purified water into the diffuser and then add your oil blend.
3. Turn on the diffuser and enjoy.

Focus and concentrate.

Supplies that you will need:

Rosemary Essential Oil

Lemon Essential Oil

Glass dram that is equipped with a spout for blending

Purified Water

Directions for blending:

1. In order to prepare this blend properly, you will need to have a glass dram to use for preparation prior to placing it in the diffuser. Start with the Lemon and Rosemary oil applying 4 drops into the dram.
2. Pour the purified water into the diffuser and then add your oil blend.
3. Turn on the diffuser and enjoy.

Chapter 13: Easy to Follow Recipes for Multiple Needs

Hormone

What you will need:

- Water
- Rosemary Aromatic Oil (20 D)
- Lavender Aromatic Oil (20 D)
- Ylang-Ylang Aromatic Oil (10 D)
- Rose Otto Aromatic Oil (10 D)
- Geranium Aromatic Oil (20 D)
- Peppermint Aromatic Oil (10 D)
- Chamomile (Roman) Aromatic Oil (10 D)
- Glass dram

Directions for blending:

5. Blend all the oils together in the order of the number of drops per oil.
6. Next, add the oils to a diffuser along with the purified water.

7. Turn the diffuser on and allow it to be set on a timer of 15 minutes on and 1 hour off.

What you will need:

- Lavender Aromatic Oil (5 D)
- Aloe Vera Gel
- Peppermint Aromatic Oil (5 D)
- Glass dram
- Water
- Spray bottle (glass)

Directions for blending:

5. Blend all the oils together in the glass dram. Twirl the dram around to blend it properly.
6. Next, pour the oils into 1 tsp Aloe Vera gel and 1 cup of distilled water.
7. Pour all of this into the spray bottle making sure it is glass.
8. Use the spray bottle to spritz your face when needed.

What you will need:

- Ylang-Ylang Aromatic Oil (5 D)
- Clary Sage Aromatic Oil (10 D)
- Bergamot Aromatic Oil (5 D)
- Rose Otto Aromatic Oil (10 D)
- Sandalwood Aromatic Oil (5 D)
- Geranium Aromatic Oil (5 D)
- Coconut Oil-Fractionated
- Glass dram
- 10-ml rollerball container

Directions for blending:

5. Blend the oils in order of the most drops to the least and then twirl the dram to incorporate them together.
6. Place the blended oils in the container with the rollerball and add the coconut oil.
7. Massage this blend into your feet, ankles, wrists and lower stomach once a day.

Digestion

What you will need:

- Carrier Oil
- Ginger Aromatic Oil (10 D)
- Peppermint Aromatic Oil (10 D)
- Chamomile Aromatic Oil (10 D)
- Glass dram

Directions for blending:

4. Blend the oils in order of the most drops to the least and then twirl the dram to incorporate them together.
5. Then, pour this oil blend into the bottle with the carrier oil that helps with nausea.
6. Sniff this blend as much as you need to help you with alleviating the feeling of nausea.

Increase immunity

What you will need:

- Water
- Rosemary Aromatic Oil (2 D)
- Cinnamon Aromatic Oil (2 D)
- Clove Aromatic Oil (2 D)
- Wild Orange Aromatic Oil (2 D)
- Eucalyptus Aromatic Oil (2 D)
- Glass dram

Directions for blending:

1. Blend all the oils together in the order of the number of drops per oil.
2. Next, add the oils to a diffuser along with the purified water.
3. Turn the diffuser on and allow it to be set on a timer of 15 minutes on and 1 hour off.

What you will need:

- Water
- On Guard Aromatic Oil (4 D) (DoTerra Brand)
- Oregano Aromatic Oil (2 D)
- Lavender Aromatic Oil (3 D)
- Glass dram

Directions for blending:

1. Blend all the oils together in the order of the number of drops per oil.
2. Next, add the oils to a diffuser along with the purified water.
3. Turn the diffuser on and allow it to be set on a timer of 15 minutes on and 1 hour off.

What you will need:

- Water
- On guard Aromatic Oil (5 D) (DoTerra blend)
- Tea Tree Aromatic Oil (1 D)
- Lemon Aromatic Oil (2 D)
- Glass dram

Directions for blending:

1. Blend all the oils together in the order of the number of drops per oil.
2. Next, add the oils to a diffuser along with the purified water.
3. Turn the diffuser on and allow it to be set on a timer of 15 minutes on and 1 hour off.

What you will need:

- Water
- Rosemary Aromatic Oil (1 D)
- Lime Aromatic Oil (1 D)
- Eucalyptus Aromatic Oil (2 D)
- Lemon Aromatic Oil (2 D)
- Peppermint Aromatic Oil (2 D)
- Clove Aromatic Oil (1 D)
- Glass dram

Directions for blending:

1. Blend all the oils together in the order of the number of drops per oil.
2. Next, add the oils to a diffuser along with the purified water.
3. Turn the diffuser on and allow it to be set on a timer of 15 minutes on and 1 hour off.

What you will need:

- Water
- Rosemary Aromatic Oil (2 D)
- Cinnamon Aromatic Oil (2 D)
- Wild Orange Aromatic Oil (2 D)
- Eucalyptus Aromatic Oil (2 D)
- Clove Aromatic Oil (2 D)
- Glass dram

Directions for blending:

1. Blend all the oils together in the order of the number of drops per oil.
2. Next, add the oils to a diffuser along with the purified water.
3. Turn the diffuser on and allow it to be set on a timer of 15 minutes on and 1 hour off.

What you will need:

- Water
- Juniper Berry Aromatic Oil (3 D)
- Lavender Aromatic Oil (3 D)
- Chamomile (Roman) Aromatic Oil (3 D)
- Glass dram

Directions for blending:

1. Blend all the oils together in the order of the number of drops per oil.
2. Next, add the oils to a diffuser along with the purified water.
3. Turn the diffuser on and allow it to be set on a timer of 15 minutes on and 1 hour off.

What you will need:

- Water
- Cedarwood Aromatic Oil (4D)
- Glass dram
- Lavender Aromatic Oil (3D)

Directions for blending:

1. Blend all the oils together in the order of the number of drops per oil.
2. Next, add the oils to a diffuser along with the purified water.
3. Turn the diffuser on and allow it to be set on a timer of 15 minutes on and 1 hour off.

What you will need:

- Water
- Vetiver Aromatic Oil (3 D)
- Frankincense Aromatic Oil (2 D)
- Lavender Aromatic Oil (3 D)
- Glass dram

Directions for blending:

1. Blend all the oils together in the order of the number of drops per oil.
2. Next, add the oils to a diffuser along with the purified water.
3. Turn the diffuser on and allow it to be set on a timer of 15 minutes on and 1 hour off.

What you will need:

- Water
- Vetiver Aromatic Oil (2 D)
- Balance Aromatic Oil (3 D) (DoTerra blend)
- Lavender Aromatic Oil (2 D)
- Chamomile (Roman) Aromatic Oil (3 D)
- Glass dram

Directions for blending:

1. Blend all the oils together in the order of the number of drops per oil.
2. Next, add the oils to a diffuser along with the purified water.
3. Turn the diffuser on and allow it to be set on a timer of 15 minutes on and 1 hour off.

What you will need:

- Allspice Aromatic Oil (10D)
- Glass dram
- Melissa Aromatic Oils (10D)
- Water

Directions for blending:

1. Blend the oils in order of the most drops to the least and then twirl the dram to incorporate them together.
2. Then apply the oils to the diffuser with the water and turn it on.
3. Allow it to run for 15 minutes and sit for 1 hour.

PMS

What you will need:

- Peppermint Aromatic Oil (5D)
- Glass rollerball
- Cypress Aromatic Oil (4D)
- Jojoba
- Lavender Aromatic Oil (3D)
- Glass dram

Directions for blending:

6. Blend the oils in the order of the most drops to the least and then twirl the dram to incorporate them together.
7. Next, pour the jojoba oil and the blend together and twirl them to blend properly.
8. Use this oil to massage your lower stomach and relieve cramping once per day.

What you will need:

- Geranium Aromatic Oil (1 D)
- Avocado oil
- Clary Sage Aromatic Oil (3 D)
- Lavender Aromatic Oil (2 D)
- Glass dram
- 10-ml glass container

Directions for blending:

6. Blend the oils in the order of the most drops to the least and then twirl the dram to incorporate them together.
7. Next, blend the oils with the avocado oil and place the lid of the rollerball on the container.
8. Use this to massage into your lower stomach for cramps.

What you will need:

- Epsom Salt
- Lavender Aromatic Oil (10 D)
- Whole Milk
- Lemon Aromatic Oil (10 D)
- Glass dram
- Peppermint Aromatic Oil (10 D)

Directions for blending:

5. Blend the oils in the order of the most drops to the least and then twirl the dram to incorporate them together.
6. Run a hot bath, pour in 2 cups of the Epsom salt and let it soak in.
7. Then, pour your aromatic oil blend into the bath and swirl it to blend in with the water.
8. Sit in your bath for a relaxing 15 minutes and enjoy the therapeutic benefits.

Fertility

What you will need:

- Rollerball
- Carrier oil (1 tbsp)
- Geranium Aromatic Oil (2 D)
- Basil Aromatic Oil (2 D)
- Cypress Aromatic Oil (2 D)

Directions for blending:

1. Blend the oils in order of the most drops to the least and then twirl the dram to incorporate them together.
2. Place the blended oils into the rollerball with the carrier oil and twirl for blending properly.
3. Use the rollerball to rub on your abdomen twice a day.

What you will need:

- Rollerball
- Carrier oil (2-oz)
- Clary Sage Aromatic Oil (25 D)
- Basil Aromatic Oil (10 D)
- Marjoram Aromatic Oil (15 D)
- Lavender Aromatic Oil (5 D)
- Ylang-Ylang Aromatic Oil (2 D)
- Geranium Aromatic Oil (15 D)
- Cypress Aromatic Oil (2 D)

Directions for blending:

1. Blend the oils in the order of the most drops to the least and then twirl the dram to incorporate them together.
2. Place the blended oils into the rollerball with the carrier oil and twirl for blending properly.
3. Use the rollerball to rub on the underneath of your feet and inside of the ankles for fertility relief for men.

What you will need:

- Rollerball
- Carrier oil (1 tbsp)
- Frankincense Aromatic Oil (10 D)
- Clary Sage Aromatic Oil (25 D)
- Eucalyptus Aromatic Oil (5 D)
- Lavender Aromatic Oil (5 D)
- Geranium Aromatic Oil (15 D)
- Ylang-Ylang Aromatic Oil (3 D)
- Basil Aromatic Oil (10 D)
- Marjoram Aromatic Oil (15 D)
- Cypress Aromatic Oil (2 D)

Directions for blending:

1. Blend the oils in the order of the most drops to the least and then twirl the dram to incorporate them together.
2. Place the blended oils into the rollerball with the carrier oil and twirl for blending properly.
3. Use the rollerball to rub on the bottom of your feet twice per day.

What you will need:

- Thyme Aromatic Oil (3 D)
- Carrier oil (1 tbsp)
- Marjoram Aromatic Oil (3 D)

Directions for blending:

1. Blend the oils in the order of the most drops to the least and then twirl the dram to incorporate them together.
2. Place the blended oils into the rollerball with the carrier oil and twirl for blending properly.
3. Use the rollerball to rub on your liver prior to bedtime.

What you will need:

- Frankincense Aromatic Oil (2D)

Directions for blending:

1. Drop 2 drops of Frankincense underneath your tongue first thing in the morning and last thing before bed. Make sure the oils are graded for food.

What you will need:

- Rollerball
- Carrier oil (1 tbsp)
- Geranium Aromatic Oil (2 D)

Directions for blending:

1. Blend the oils in the order of the most drops to the least and then twirl the dram to incorporate them together.
2. Place the blended oils into the rollerball with the carrier oil and twirl for blending properly.
3. Use the rollerball to rub on your adrenal glands every morning.

What you will need:

- Rollerball
- Carrier oil - coconut oil (1 tbsp)
- Cypress Aromatic Oil (3 D)
- Chamomile (Roman) Aromatic Oil (3 D)
- Frankincense Aromatic Oil (3 D)

Directions for blending:

1. Blend the oils in the order of the most drops to the least and then twirl the dram to incorporate them together.
2. Place the blended oils into the rollerball with the carrier oil and twirl for blending properly.
3. Use the rollerball to rub on the underneath of your feet first thing in the AM and last thing in the PM.

What you will need:

- Rollerball
- Carrier oil (1 tbsp)
- Sandalwood Aromatic Oil (2 D)
- Basil Aromatic Oil (2 D)
- Goldenrod Aromatic Oil (2 D)

Directions for blending:

1. Blend the oils in the order of the most drops to the least and then twirl the dram to incorporate them together.
2. Place the blended oils into the rollerball with the carrier oil and twirl for blending properly.
3. Use the rollerball to rub on the inside of the man's ankles, sacral vertebrae, and wrists 2 times per day.

What you will need:

- Rollerball
- Carrier oil (1 tbsp)
- Clary Sage Aromatic Oil (6 D)

Directions for blending:

1. Blend the oils in the order of the most drops to the least and then twirl the dram to incorporate them together.
2. Place the blended oils into the rollerball with the carrier oil and twirl for blending properly.
3. Use the rollerball to rub on the abdomen near the mons pubis and the ankles 2 times per day.

Pregnancy

What you will need:

- Rollerball
- Carrier oil-Almond oil (3 tbsp)
- Sweet Marjoram Aromatic Oil (1 D)
- Juniper Berry Aromatic Oil (1 D)
- Cypress Aromatic Oil (1 D)
- Frankincense Carterii Aromatic Oil (1 D)

Directions for blending:

1. Blend the oils in the order of the most drops to the least and then twirl the dram to incorporate them together.
2. Place the blended oils into the rollerball with the carrier oil and twirl for blending properly.
3. Use the rollerball to rub on the feet and legs 2 times per day.

What you will need:

- Coco butter-Melted (2 tsp)
- Lavender Aromatic Oil (1 D)
- Frankincense Aromatic Oil (1 D)
- Chamomile (Roman) Aromatic Oil (1 D)

Directions for blending:

1. Blend the oils in the order of the most drops to the least and then twirl the dram to incorporate them together.
2. Place the coco butter in your hand and pour the blend on top. Rub your hands to blend the oil with the butter.
3. Use the butter to massage your belly for skin that is silky smooth.

What you will need:

- Bergamot Aromatic Oil (2D)
- Orange Aromatic Oil (2D)
- Ylang-Ylang Aromatic Oil (2D)
- Water

Directions for blending:

1. Blend the oils in the order of the most drops to the least and then twirl the dram to incorporate them together.
2. Pour the water into the diffuser and then add in your blend.
3. Turn the diffuser on for 15 minutes then let it sit for 1 hour.

What you will need:

- Water
- Ginger root Aromatic Oil (1 D)
- Greek Lavender Aromatic Oil (1 D)
- Black Pepper Aromatic Oil (1 D)
- Grapefruit Aromatic Oil (1 D)

Directions for blending:

1. Blend the oils in the order of the most drops to the least and then twirl the dram to incorporate them together.
2. Pour the water into the diffuser and then add the blended oils.
3. Turn the diffuser on and let it run for 15 minutes. Then turn it off and let it sit for 1 hour.

Menopause

What you will need:

- Carrier Oil-Grapeseed (2 oz.)
- Clary sage Aromatic Oil (2 D)
- Angelica Aromatic Oil (1 D)
- Jasmine Aromatic Oil (1 D)
- Lemon Aromatic Oil (6 D)
- Geranium Aromatic Oil (5 D)

Directions for blending:

1. Blend the oils in the order of the most drops to the least and then twirl the dram to incorporate them together.
2. Blend the oil blend with the carrier oil and place the rollerball lid on the bottle. Twirl the bottle to blend properly.
3. Apply this blend every day or pour into your hot bath.

What you will need:

- Clary Sage Aromatic Oil (30 D)
- Thyme Greek Lavender Aromatic Oil (30 D)
- Ylang-Ylang Aromatic Oil (30 D)
- Evening Primrose Aromatic Oil (1 oz.)

Directions for blending:

1. Blend the oils in the order of the most drops to the least and then twirl the dram to incorporate them together.
2. Pour the Evening Primrose into the oil blend and then twirl to blend properly.
3. Apply to a bath or a small amount on your neck in the morning and night time.

What you will need:

- Water-distilled (3 oz)
- Peppermint Aromatic Oil (8 D)
- Clary Sage Aromatic Oil (8 D)
- Witch Hazel (1 oz.)
- Chamomile (Roman) Aromatic Oil (8 D)
- Grapefruit Aromatic Oil (1 D)

Directions for blending:

1. Blend the oils in the order of the most drops to the least and then twirl the dram to incorporate them together.
2. Pour the blend into a spray bottle and add the witch hazel.
3. Shake and spray on your neck, back, and torso if you experience a hot flash. Do not get near eyes.

What you will need:

- Water-distilled (3 c)
- Eucalyptus Aromatic Oil (5 D)
- Peppermint Aromatic Oil (5 D)

Directions for blending:

1. Blend the oils in the order of the most drops to the least and then twirl the dram to incorporate them together.
2. Place a washcloth or towel in the water with the oils. Squeeze out the water.
3. Roll the towel like a swiss roll and freeze in the freezer.
4. Apply to the chest, forehead, neck, and other parts when you are having hot sweats.

What you will need:

- Ylang-Ylang Aromatic Oil (3 D)
- Carrier Oil-Jojoba (1 tsp)
- Orange Aromatic Oil (1 D)

Directions for blending:

1. Blend the oils in the order of the most drops to the least and then twirl the dram to incorporate them together.
2. Then blend the oil blend with the carrier oil.
3. Using it as a lotion, apply it to the thyroid glands that are located on the throat. Then apply to the wrists, as well as the neck. This will increase your libido which helps relax the atmosphere.

What you will need:

- Ylang-Ylang Aromatic Oil (3D)
- Carrier Oil-Jojoba (1tsp)
- Orange Aromatic Oil (1D)
- Sandalwood Aromatic Oil (1D)

Directions for blending:

1. Blend the oils in the order of the most drops to the least and then twirl the dram to incorporate them together.
2. Then blend the oil blend with the carrier oil.
3. Using it as a lotion, apply it to the thyroid glands that are located on the throat. Then apply to the wrists, as well as the neck. This will increase your libido which helps relax the atmosphere.

What you will need:

- Neroli Aromatic Oil (10 D)
- Frankincense Aromatic Oil (10 D)
- Chamomile (Roman) Aromatic Oil (5 D)
- St. John's Wort (0.333 c)
- Carrier Oil-Jojoba (1 tsp)
- Lavender Aromatic Oil (7 D)
- Calendula (0.25 C)
- Comfrey Leaf (0.333 C)
- Orange Aromatic Oil (1 D)

Directions for blending:

1. Melt your wax in a boiler that is doubled.
2. Once it reaches a specific texture, add in the 3 carrier oils.
3. Stir to blend
4. Blend the oils in the order of the most drops to the least and then twirl the dram to incorporate them together. Add them to the cooled wax mix.
5. Pour into jars and let them solidify.
6. Store in dry and cool locations.
7. Give them 2 hours to solidify and then use as a salve for your dryness down there.

What you will need:

- Clary sage Aromatic Oil (2 D)
- Marjoram Aromatic Oil (2 D)
- Geranium Aromatic Oil (1 D)
- Lavender Aromatic Oil (2 D)
- Chamomile (Roman) Aromatic Oil (1 D)
- Ylang-Ylang Aromatic Oil (2 D)
- Carrier Oil-Evening Primrose (15 ml)

Directions for blending:

1. Blend the oils in the order of the most drops to the least and then twirl the dram to incorporate them together.
2. Then blend the oil blend with the carrier oil.
3. Using it as a lotion, apply it to the abdomen.
4. Take time to massage this blend into your skin so that you will have fewer mood swings and be less irritable.

What you will need:

- Peppermint Aromatic Oil (3 D)
- Grapefruit Aromatic Oil (3 D)
- Basil Aromatic Oil (3 D)
- Water-distilled

Directions for blending:

1. Blend the oils in the order of the most drops to the least and then twirl the dram to incorporate them together.
2. Add to the diffuser with the water.
3. Turn on the diffuser and allow it to run for 15 minutes. Then let it sit for 1 hour.

What you will need:

- Lavender Aromatic Oil (15 D)
- Coconut oil-fractionated (10 ml)
- Wild Orange Aromatic Oil (5 D)
- Vetiver Aromatic Oil (10 D)
- Frankincense Aromatic Oil (5 D)
- Ylang-Ylang Aromatic Oil (5 D)

Directions for blending:

1. Blend the oils in the order of the most drops to the least and then twirl the dram to incorporate them together.
2. Add the blended oils with the coconut oil in the rollerball.
3. Use this oil to massage nightly on your feet as well as on your neck for better sleep.

Candida

What you will need:

- Tea Tree Aromatic Oil (10 D)
- Coconut oil (1 tbsp)

Directions for blending:

1. Wash your feet prior to using this blend.
2. Blend the oil with the coconut and then apply to your feet.
3. Once applied, slide a sock over the foot to help it soak in.
4. Do this prior to going to bed.

What you will need:

- Tea Tree Aromatic Oil (8 D)
- Water-distilled (2 c)
- Listerine (0.50 c)
- Epsom Salt (1 c)
- Witch Hazel (0.50 c)
- White Vinegar (1 c)

Directions for blending:

1. Wash your feet prior to using this blend.
2. Blend the ingredients together in a basin.
3. Soak your feet in this basin for 30 minutes or more.
4. Use nightly to block infections from forming.
5. Dry your feet completely and apply first the salve that was mentioned.

What you will need:

- Cinnamon Aromatic Oil (3 D)
- Water-distilled (2 c)
- Listerine (0.50 c)
- Epsom Salt (1 c)
- Witch Hazel (0.50 c)
- White Vinegar (1 c)

Directions for blending:

1. Wash your feet prior to using this blend.
2. Blend the ingredients together in a basin.
3. Soak your feet in this basin for 30 minutes or more.
4. Use nightly to block infections from forming.
5. Dry your feet completely and apply first the salve that was mentioned.

What you will need:

- Clove Aromatic Oil (3 D)
- Water-distilled (2 c)
- Listerine (0.50 c)
- Epsom Salt (1 c)
- Witch Hazel (0.50 c)
- White Vinegar (1 c)

Directions for blending:

1. Wash your feet prior to using this blend.
2. Blend the ingredients together in a basin.
3. Soak your feet in this basin for 30 minutes or more.
4. Use nightly to block infections from forming.
5. Dry your feet completely and apply first the salve that was mentioned.

What you will need:

- Oregano Aromatic Oil (3 D)
- Water-distilled (2 c)
- Listerine (0.50 c)
- Epsom Salt (1 c)
- Witch Hazel (0.50 c)
- White Vinegar (1 c)

Directions for blending:

1. Wash your feet prior to using this blend.
2. Blend the ingredients together in a basin.
3. Soak your feet in this basin for 30 minutes or more.
4. Use nightly to block infections from forming.
5. Dry your feet completely and apply first the salve that was mentioned.

Emotional Blends

What you will need:

- Peppermint Aromatic Oil (4 D)
- Rosemary Aromatic Oil (2 D)
- Cinnamon Aromatic Oil (4 D)
- Water-distilled

Directions for blending:

1. Blend the oils in the order of the most drops to the least and then twirl the dram to incorporate them together.
2. Add to the diffuser with the water.
3. Turn on the diffuser and allow it to run for 15 minutes. Then let it sit for 1 hour.

What you will need:

- Peppermint Aromatic Oil (3 D)
- Rosemary Aromatic Oil (3 D)
- Frankincense Aromatic Oil (3 D)
- Water-distilled

Directions for blending:

1. Blend the oils in the order of the most drops to the least and then twirl the dram to incorporate them together.
2. Add to the diffuser with the water.
3. Turn on the diffuser and allow it to run for 15 minutes. Then let it sit for 1 hour.

What you will need:

- Frankincense Aromatic Oil (2 D)
- Balance Aromatic Oil (4 D) (DoTerra Blend)
- Vetiver Aromatic Oil (2 D)
- Water-distilled

Directions for blending:

1. Blend the oils in the order of the most drops to the least and then twirl the dram to incorporate them together.
2. Add to the diffuser with the water.
3. Turn on the diffuser and allow it to run for 15 minutes. Then let it sit for 1 hour.

What you will need:

- Lemon Aromatic Oil (2 D)
- Grapefruit Aromatic Oil (2 D)
- Rosemary Aromatic Oil (1 D)
- Peppermint Aromatic Oil (2 D)
- Basil Aromatic Oil (1 D)
- Lavender Aromatic Oil (2 D)
- Water-distilled

Directions for blending:

1. Blend the oils in the order of the most drops to the least and then twirl the dram to incorporate them together.
2. Add to the diffuser with the water.
3. Turn on the diffuser and allow it to run for 15 minutes. Then let it sit for 1 hour.

What you will need:

- Ylang-Ylang Aromatic Oil (2 D)
- Clary Sage Aromatic Oil (3 D)
- Marjoram Aromatic Oil (1 D)
- Lavender Aromatic Oil (4 D)
- Water-distilled

Directions for blending:

1. Blend the oils in the order of the most drops to the least and then twirl the dram to incorporate them together.
2. Add to the diffuser with the water.
3. Turn on the diffuser and allow it to run for 15 minutes. Then let it sit for 1 hour.

What you will need:

- Frankincense Aromatic Oil (4 D)
- Balance Aromatic Oil (4 D) (DoTerra Blend)
- Water-distilled

Directions for blending:

1. Blend the oils in the order of the most drops to the least and then twirl the dram to incorporate them together.
2. Add to the diffuser with the water.
3. Turn on the diffuser and allow it to run for 15 minutes. Then let it sit for 1 hour.

What you will need:

- Ylang-Ylang Aromatic Oil (4 D)
- Lavender Aromatic Oil (3 D)
- Chamomile (Roman) Aromatic Oil (2 D)
- Water-distilled

Directions for blending:

1. Blend the oils in the order of the most drops to the least and then twirl the dram to incorporate them together.
2. Add to the diffuser with the water.
3. Turn on the diffuser and allow it to run for 15 minutes. Then let it sit for 1 hour.

Better day Blends

What you will need:

- Elevation Aromatic Oil (3 D)
- Frankincense Aromatic Oil (3 D)
- Bergamot Aromatic Oil (3 D)
- Water-distilled

Directions for blending:

1. Blend the oils in the order of the most drops to the least and then twirl the dram to incorporate them together.
2. Add to the diffuser with the water.
3. Turn on the diffuser and allow it to run for 15 minutes. Then let it sit for 1 hour.

What you will need:

- Wild Orange Aromatic Oil (2 D)
- Lavender Aromatic Oil (4 D)
- Cedarwood Aromatic Oil (2 D)
- Water-distilled

Directions for blending:

1. Blend the oils in the order of the most drops to the least and then twirl the dram to incorporate them together.
2. Add to the diffuser with the water.
3. Turn on the diffuser and allow it to run for 15 minutes. Then let it sit for 1 hour.

What you will need:

- Peppermint Aromatic Oil (4 D)
- Rosemary Aromatic Oil (2 D)
- Ylang-Ylang Aromatic Oil (1 D)
- Cinnamon Aromatic Oil (4 D)
- Water-distilled

Directions for blending:

1. Blend the oils in the order of the most drops to the least and then twirl the dram to incorporate them together.
2. Add to the diffuser with the water.
3. Turn on the diffuser and allow it to run for 15 minutes. Then let it sit for 1 hour.

What you will need:

- Patchouli Aromatic Oil (3 D)
- Ylang-Ylang Aromatic Oil (3 D)
- Bergamot Aromatic Oil (3 D)
- Water-distilled

Directions for blending:

1. Blend the oils in the order of the most drops to the least and then twirl the dram to incorporate them together.
2. Add to the diffuser with the water.
3. Turn on the diffuser and allow it to run for 15 minutes. Then let it sit for 1 hour.

What you will need:

- Vetiver Aromatic Oil (2 D)
- Lemon Aromatic Oil (1 D)
- Lavender Aromatic Oil (4 D)
- Clary Sage Aromatic Oil (1 D)
- Water-distilled

Directions for blending:

1. Blend the oils in the order of the most drops to the least and then twirl the dram to incorporate them together.
2. Add to the diffuser with the water.
3. Turn on the diffuser and allow it to run for 15 minutes. Then let it sit for 1 hour.

Mood Elevation

What you will need:

- Lavender Aromatic Oil (3 D)
- Clary Sage Aromatic Oil (2 D)
- Geranium Aromatic Oil (3 D)
- Chamomile (Roman) Aromatic Oil (2 D)
- Ylang-Ylang Aromatic Oil (2 D)
- Water-distilled

Directions for blending:

1. Blend the oils in the order of the most drops to the least and then twirl the dram to incorporate them together.
2. Add to the diffuser with the water.
3. Turn on the diffuser and allow it to run for 15 minutes. Then let it sit for 1 hour.

What you will need:

- Lime Aromatic Oil (3 D)
- Lavender Aromatic Oil (3 D)
- Mandarin Aromatic Oil (3 D)
- Water-distilled

Directions for blending:

1. Blend the oils in the order of the most drops to the least and then twirl the dram to incorporate them together.
2. Add to the diffuser with the water.
3. Turn on the diffuser and allow it to run for 15 minutes. Then let it sit for 1 hour.

What you will need:

- Peppermint Aromatic Oil (3 D)
- Rosemary Aromatic Oil (3 D)
- Lemon Aromatic Oil (3 D)
- Water-distilled

Directions for blending:

1. Blend the oils in the order of the most drops to the least and then twirl the dram to incorporate them together.
2. Add to the diffuser with the water.
3. Turn on the diffuser and allow it to run for 15 minutes. Then let it sit for 1 hour.

What you will need:

- Peppermint Aromatic Oil (3 D)
- Rosemary Aromatic Oil (3 D)
- Grapefruit Aromatic Oil (2 D)
- Water-distilled

Directions for blending:

1. Blend the oils in the order of the most drops to the least and then twirl the dram to incorporate them together.
2. Add to the diffuser with the water.
3. Turn on the diffuser and allow it to run for 15 minutes. Then let it sit for 1 hour.

What you will need:

- Cinnamon Aromatic Oil (2 D)
- Wild Orange Aromatic Oil (3 D)
- Frankincense Aromatic Oil (3 D)
- Water-distilled

Directions for blending:

1. Blend the oils in the order of the most drops to the least and then twirl the dram to incorporate them together.
2. Add to the diffuser with the water.
3. Turn on the diffuser and allow it to run for 15 minutes. Then let it sit for 1 hour.

What you will need:

- Peppermint Aromatic Oil (4 D)
- Wild Orange Aromatic Oil (4 D)
- Water-distilled

Directions for blending:

1. Blend the oils in the order of the most drops to the least and then twirl the dram to incorporate them together.
2. Add to the diffuser with the water.
3. Turn on the diffuser and allow it to run for 15 minutes. Then let it sit for 1 hour.

What you will need:

- Bergamot Aromatic Oil (3 D)
- Lavender Aromatic Oil (3 D)
- Geranium Aromatic Oil (2 D)
- Water-distilled

Directions for blending:

1. Blend the oils in the order of the most drops to the least and then twirl the dram to incorporate them together.
2. Add to the diffuser with the water.
3. Turn on the diffuser and allow it to run for 15 minutes. Then let it sit for 1 hour.

What you will need:

- Peppermint Aromatic Oil (2 D)
- Wild Orange Aromatic Oil (2 D)
- Frankincense Aromatic Oil (2 D)
- Lime Aromatic Oil (2 D)
- Water-distilled

Directions for blending:

1. Blend the oils in order of the most drops to the least and then twirl the dram to incorporate them together.
2. Add to the diffuser with the water.
3. Turn on the diffuser and allow it to run for 15 minutes. Then let it sit for 1 hour.

Alternative Remedies for insects

Insect bites spray

Directions for blending:

- Lemon Aromatic Oils (1 D)
- Tea Tree Aromatic Oils (2 D)
- Juniper berries Aromatic Oil (2 D)
- Spray bottle-Glass
- Borage Aromatic Oil (1 tsp)
- Glass dram
- Carrier oils-jojoba or almond

Directions for blending:

1. Blend the oils in the order of the most drops to the least and then twirl the dram to incorporate them together.
2. Then, mix the Borage with the other oils in the spray bottle.
3. Roll oils in the palms of your hands. This will blend them together properly.
4. After you have placed the blended Aromatic oils into the spray bottle, you can begin to use this spray to ward off insects.

5. Insects can be very aggravating and this will help you to get rid of the itch and keep them away.

To apply:

Prior to using this on your child, verify that they are not allergic to the blend or any of the individual oils. After you have verified this, you are good to use it on a daily basis as a preventative spray, as a way to comb the hair after an infestation, and in your shampoo for the whole house. You can also spray all of your furniture with this oil blend. It will keep the bugs at bay, and we all know how quickly you can pick these little annoying bugs up when you have children in school or daycare. I know that this has saved my household a time or two and I live by this recipe. It is not only easy to use but also saves you all that money which it would cost to pick up a lice treatment kit in the grocery store, especially since the kits are $20 or more dollars and the number of oils you use for this recipe would cost you less in the long run.

Lice Be-gone

Supplies that you will need:

- Ginger Aromatic Oils (5 D)
- Lavender Aromatic Oils (5 D)
- Carrier oils- your choice
- Walnut Aromatic Oil (1 tsp)
- Peppermint Aromatic Oil (5 D)
- Glass storage bowl
- Glass dram

Directions for blending:

1. Blend the oils in the order of the most drops to the least and then twirl the dram to incorporate them together.
2. Then, blend the oil blend with the carrier oils and place them in a spray bottle of use as a salve.
3. Once the aromatic oils are blended, you can use this treatment to kill head lice. This will also prevent them from coming back.
4. Store your oil blend in a glass container that is sealable and use it every week to protect against these annoying little bugs.

5. Coat the hair with this blend like a hair mask and let it sit overnight.

Conclusion

Thanks for making it through to the end of *Essential Oils: Ancient Medicine*!

I bet you are pleased with your purchase.

Of course, who would not be pleased with a book that not only teaches you what essential oils are but also how to use them to your own advantage? I know that you are ready to start calculating your own blends—and thanks to your decision to download this book, you are able to do that. I have not only taken you from a beginner essential oil user, but I have given you an aromatherapist-level knowledge on the essence of an essential oil and the process by which you can create your own blends.

With all the details contained in this book, you should have no problem developing your own blends and reaching the results that you are craving. Essential oils are created from your favorite plants—and by harvesting them and using them for alternative remedies, you are able to experience earth in a different way. The use of essential oils has been employed since prior to the Egyptian society. And now, you are blessed with so many resources that you can begin to harness this power and knowledge that the Egyptians knew all along.

Now that you have learned this technique, I have been able to add some teaching class for me.

Essential oils are a wonderful alternative to modern medicine for those that wish to only use what has come from the Earth. In ancient times, it was believed that witches used essential oils to hex people—but this simply was not true. Essential oils have been healing families and people since 6000 years ago.

Knowing the history of any practice helps you in fully utilizing it, which is why it's important to know that essential oils have a labyrinth of magical practices and medicinal uses through all of the world's cultures. In order to know the history, you need to start out with the Egyptians, since they created ways for everyone to incorporate the use of essential oils into every aspect of their lives. In Egyptian times even, the servants were allowed to use this powerful alternative medication for perfumes and healing. The employment of essential oils is not solely stemmed in disorder and drugs—it can also be instrumental to the improvement of life.

Since several cultures believe in the magic of plants, it is solely natural that the planet would return to the conclusion that essential oils are helpful and enhance our lives and health. With the employment of rituals, cooking, and drugs within the history of each culture, knowing what essential oils are best for you is as easy as learning a book—like this one.

I know that after reading this book, you are ready to start purchasing only the best oils for your family. If that is the case, then check out www.planttherapy.com and www.mountainroseherb.com. They have been providing some of the purest and most authentic oils for a long time.

In order to check the purity of any oil, simply do a test that is designed to check the oils' lasting effects. If the oil you are using is bloated on a piece of watercolor paper and is still visible or aromatic after 48 hours, then it is not authentic. This oil would have been altered and blended with another chemical to help it last longer. If it is not still visible or aromatic, then you have found a pure and authentic oil to use.

Now that you know how to use oil, how to test their purity, and what to use them for, you should be able to start helping your family feel better and look better. We are all looking for better ways to care for our families. And by using essences that are derived from plants, you can begin to take that holistic journey into the alternative medicine world.

Aromatherapy is one of the best ways to calm the mind, get better sleep, and alleviate many of your ailments. I hope that you have found this book to be helpful for your aromatherapy needs and that you are able to utilize these recipes as I do every day.

Enjoy the recipes for:

- The elevation of moods.
- Having a better day.
- Healing those emotional disturbances.
- Candida and how to cure and prevent it.
- Ways to kick menopause in the butt.
- How to handle all the things that come with pregnancy.
- How to increase your chances of fertility for both you and him.
- Handling PMS like a champion.
- Increasing your immunity so that you do not get sick.
- Helping with your digestion.
- And last but not least, increasing your hormone levels for optimal health.

I have also included:

- The history behind the use of these essences which are derived from plants.
- How the English used them during the Renaissance.
- The ways that we went from not bathing to bathing due to the use of essence.
- How the word about essences was spread throughout the world.
- How Lavender oil was found to cure burns.
- The oldest known documentation on the use of essences.
- How Aromatherapy was coined.
- The original jobs of a pharmacist.
- How essences were mainstreamed and allowed for common people to purchase and use them.

I hope that is enough information for you to understand how useful this book is for you.

Thanks!

CPSIA information can be obtained
at www.ICGtesting.com
Printed in the USA
BVHW081212091120
592845BV00013B/1212